Mentoring
Health Science Professionals

Sana Loue, JD, PhD, MPH, MSSA, is a professor in the School of Medicine of Case Western Reserve University, with a primary appointment in the Department of Epidemiology and Biostatistics and secondary appointments in the Departments of Psychiatry, Bioethics, and Global Health. Dr. Loue holds a law degree, doctoral degrees in epidemiology and in medical anthropology, and master's degrees in public health, social work, and secondary education. Her research focuses on HIV/AIDS, family violence, and mental illness in minority and marginalized communities in the United States and overseas. She is an author of more than 75 peer-reviewed articles and 60 chapters, and has authored or edited more than 25 books and produced 7 educational/ training videos. She has mentored more than 60 health professionals at the predoctoral, postdoctoral, and faculty levels.

Mentoring
Health Science Professionals

Sana Loue, JD, PhD, MPH, MSSA

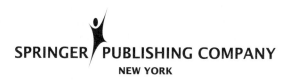

SPRINGER PUBLISHING COMPANY
NEW YORK

Springer Publishing Company, LLC
11 West 42nd Street
New York, NY 10036
www.springerpub.com

Acquisitions Editor: Sheri W. Sussman
Senior Editor: Rose Mary Piscitelli
Cover design: Joseph DePinho
Project Manager: Nandini Loganathan
Composition: S4Carlisle Publishing Services

ISBN: 978-0-8261-0476-2
E-book ISBN: 978-0-8261-0477-9

10 11 12 13/5 4 3 2 1

The author and the publisher of this Work have made every effort to use sources believed to be reliable to provide information that is accurate and compatible with the standards generally accepted at the time of publication. The author and publisher shall not be liable for any special, consequential, or exemplary damages resulting, in whole or in part, from the readers' use of, or reliance on, the information contained in this book. The publisher has no responsibility for the persistence or accuracy of URLs for external or third-party Internet Web sites referred to in this publication and does not guarantee that any content on such Web sites is, or will remain, accurate or appropriate.

Library of Congress Cataloging-in-Publication Data

Mentoring health science professionals/[edited by] Sana Loue.
    p. ; cm.
  Includes bibliographical references.
  ISBN 978-0-8261-0476-2 (softback)
1. Mentoring in medicine. I. Loue, Sana.
  [DNLM: 1. Mentors. 2. Education, Medical—methods. 3. Health Personnel. W 18]
  R834.M457 2010
  610—dc22
                                                                                    2010045890

Printed in the United States of America by Hamilton Printing

"Tell me and I'll forget; show me and I may remember; involve me and I'll understand."

Proverb

Contents

Contributors

Kathleen Clegg, MD, Case Western Reserve University School of Medicine, Cleveland, Ohio

Oscar Grusky, PhD, University of California Los Angeles, Los Angeles, California

Sarah McCue Horwitz, PhD, Stanford University, Stanford, California

Beatrice Gabriela Ioan, MD, PhD, MA, University of Medicine and Pharmacy "Gr. T. Popa," Iasi, Romania

Linda S. Lloyd, DrPH, The Institute for Palliative Medicine at San Diego Hospice, San Diego, California

Daniel J. O'Shea, BS, Public Health Services, County of San Diego, San Diego, California

Klara K. Papp, PhD, Case Western Reserve University School of Medicine, Cleveland, Ohio

Eric Rice, PhD, University of Southern California School of Social Work, Los Angeles, California

Robert Ronis, MD, MPH, Case Western Reserve University School of Medicine, Cleveland, Ohio

Richard Rudick, MD, The Cleveland Clinic Lerner College of Medicine and The Cleveland Clinic, Cleveland, Ohio

Martha Sajatovic, MD, Case Western Reserve University School of Medicine, Cleveland, Ohio

James C. Spilsbury, PhD, The Cleveland Clinic, Cleveland, Ohio

Preface

Mentoring has for a long time been deemed critical to the success of health professionals, whether as clinicians, researchers, or teachers. Successful efforts to address this need must thoughtfully consider the process, content, goals, and outcomes of the mentoring effort.

It is not possible in the space of one volume to address the many details that comprise mentoring efforts in each and every health discipline. This text seeks, instead, to provide mentors and mentees in the health professions with a blueprint for the development and evaluation of mentoring efforts. Each chapter provides the reader with an integration of the relevant published literature, while the case studies that follow provide accounts of the firsthand experiences of mentors and mentees in a variety of health professions across diverse settings.

Chapter 1 lays the foundation through a discussion of the mentoring process and the various models of mentoring that are available. This is followed with a case study by Daniel O'Shea and Linda Lloyd, who report on the successful use of multiple models of mentoring in the context of a public health department. Chapters 2 and 3, which focus on the mentoring of faculty, students, and junior professionals, draw on both theory and empirical research to highlight successful approaches and potential pitfalls. Case Study 2, authored by Sarah Horwitz and colleagues, reflects the perspective of a mentee and his mentors as he seeks to develop a successful career trajectory as a faculty member in an academic medical setting. Kathleen Clegg and colleagues focus in Case Study 3 on mentoring psychiatry residents. Each of these case studies draws from relevant literature and actual experiences during the mentoring process, providing readers with wisdom gleaned from practical experience, theory, and empirical research.

Chapter 4 focuses on issues related to diversity in the context of mentoring programs and relationships. Diversity is defined broadly here, to encompass not only race (without arguing the existence of the construct), ethnicity, and sex, but also religion, gender identity, sexual orientation, and nationality. Beatrice Ioan expands on the concepts of this chapter in her case study focusing on her experiences as an international predoctoral trainee in research ethics.

The final chapter focuses on the development and evaluation of formal mentoring programs at the institutional, programmatic, and mentor–mentee levels. The accompanying case study, authored by Eric Rice and Oscar Grusky, provides not only suggestions for the evaluation of a mentoring relationship, but also insights into the development and transformation of that relationship over time.

The process of mentoring offers immense opportunities for the development of rewarding personal and professional relationships and for the enhancement of self-knowledge. Moreover, it allows both the mentor and the mentee to engage in a continual process of learning and to look upon each day with a renewed sense of wonderment.

Sana Loue

ONE

Mentoring: Process and Models

THE EVOLVING CONCEPT OF MENTORING

It may come as a surprise to learn that the concept of mentoring dates back to Greek mythology and the time of the Egyptian pharaohs. The term itself appears to have evolved from the term *Mentor*, used in Greek mythology. Greek literature indicates that Pallas Athena transformed herself into an older man named Mentor, who served the King of Ithaca, Odysseus, also known as Ulysses (National Academy of Sciences, National Academy of Engineering, Institute of Medicine, 1997). During his absence to fight the Trojan War, King Odysseus entrusted both the care of his son Telemachus and his kingdom to Mentor (Barondess, 1995; Ramsey, Thompson, & Braithwaite, 1994; Roberts, 1999).

Perhaps the earliest record of an actual mentor is that of Imhotep (2635–2595 BC), or Imouthes in Greek. Imhotep served as a vizer or chancellor to King Djoser, who was a pharaoh during the Third Dynasty. An accomplished architect, physician, priest, and astronomer, Imhotep is perhaps best known for the design and execution of the Step Pyramid complex in Saqqara, Egypt (Kemp, 2005).

The concept of mentoring has evolved significantly since the time of Imhotep and has been subject to a variety of definitions. Initially, mentoring was believed to be unidirectional, with the benefits inuring only to the mentee from the individual serving as the mentor. The following definitions are illustrative of many others that share this perspective (Alleman, Cochran, Doverspike, & Newman, 1984; Anderson & Shannon, 1988; Blackwell, 1989; Heller & Sindelar, 1991; Lester & Johnson, 1981; Shea, 1995; Standing Committee on Postgraduate Medical and Dental Education, 1998).

> a developmental partnership through which one person shares knowledge, skills, information and perspective to foster the personal and professional growth of someone else. (American Speech-Language Hearing Association, 2007, p. 1)

> a deliberate pairing of a more skilled or experienced person with a lesser skilled or experienced one, with the agreed-on goal of having the lesser skilled person grow and develop specific competencies. (Godshalk & Sosik, 2000, pp. 299–300)

1

> a process whereby one guides, leads, supports, teaches, and challenges other individuals to facilitate their personal, educational, and professional growth and development through mutual respect and trust . . . Mentoring is viewed not only as a relationship between two individuals, but as a process. As a growth process, mentoring can be systematically planned and evaluated. (Wright-Harp & Cole, 2008, p. 8)

Increasingly, scholars are recognizing that mentoring is a bidirectional process, with responsibilities falling on both the mentor and the mentee and benefits potentially inuring to each. This more realistic perspective is reflected in the following definitions of mentoring that follow, which are also illustrative of others' similar perspectives (Allen, Poteet, Russell, & Dobbins, 1997; Burrell, Wood, Pikes, & Holliday, 2001; Galbraith & Zelenak, 1991; Healy & Welchert, 1990). (It is also reflected in Rice's and Grusky's Case Study 5, in this book, which explores their mentor–mentee relationship.)

> a developmental, empowering and nurturing relationship extending over time in which mutual sharing, learning, and growth occur . . . it is a two-way process with learning for both parties. Thus it is acknowledged that mentoring is likely to be reciprocal in that wisdom is not handed down in a one-way transaction, rather both mentor and mentee share knowledge, insight and skills. (Fielden, Davidson, & Sutherland, 2009, p. 93)

> a planned relationship between an experienced person and one who has less experience for the purpose of achieving identified outcomes . . . mentoring has been defined as a situation that promotes personal and professional development in which general well-being is enhanced, synergy is increased, new insights are gained, perspectives on the experiences is [*sic*] developed, balance is created, and ways to succeed are discovered. This results in increased productivity and creativity on the part of both parties. (Barker, 2006, p. 56, citations omitted)

> a process of teaching and learning that takes place within a long-term personal, reciprocal relationship between two [persons] positioned on different levels, with different ages, personalities, and credentials. (Smith, McAllister, & Crawford, 2001, p. 101)

All of these definitions reflect various common themes. First, the mentor has traditionally been viewed as an individual who should have greater expertise in the relevant field or discipline in comparison with the mentee. Second, mentoring is a long-term interaction between at least two individuals. Third, a goal, if not the ultimate goal, of mentoring is the professional and personal development of the mentee, including his or her development of the skills necessary to succeed in the particular field and his or her socialization into that profession.

These latter two characteristics of mentoring help to distinguish a mentoring relationship from one of patronage, consulting, counseling, or coaching, although these functions are frequently encompassed within a mentoring relationship. In contrast to these other relationships, mentoring is focused on the process and the quality of the relationship as well as the goal. In a mentoring relationship, power is shared between the mentor and the mentee, and the mentee is recognized as both the decision maker and the expert with respect to his or her future direction (Dancer, 2003). In contrast, a relationship of patronage often views the patron as the expert and is concerned primarily with the protégé's achievement and the products that the patronage yields. Unlike a mentoring relationship, a consulting relationship is by definition time limited. The consultant is perceived as the expert and, in some circumstances, may also be viewed as a decision maker (Dancer, 2003; Smith et al., 2001). Counseling is similar to consulting in that the counselor is often viewed as the expert and the relationship is unidirectional toward the mentee. Coaching is most closely aligned with mentoring. However, coaching is also to be distinguished from mentoring by its emphasis on the attainment of specified goals that are often either professional (e.g., attainment of a higher level position) or personal (e.g., weight loss) goals, rather than issues that may cross the boundaries of these domains, such as would occur in the context of a mentoring relationship (Dancer, 2003; Hargrove, 2000).

Although a relationship between a mentor and mentee bears similarities to a relationship with a role model, and a mentor may fulfill the function of a role model, there are significant differences (Gibson, 2004). An individual may have multiple role models or multiple mentors; individuals generally have fewer primary mentors than they might have role models. The relationship between an individual and a role model is typically passive and flows in only one direction, from the individual to the role model; a mentoring relationship is bidirectional (Friedman et al., 2004). While a mentor will take interest in the progress of the mentee, this is often less true of someone who is a role model. A mentoring relationship is typically a long-term one, but a role model may be relevant for a variable length of time (Gibson, 2004).

As can be seen from these definitions, the functions of the mentor can be grouped into three broad categories: (1) the provision of vocational and/or instrumental support to enhance the career of the mentee, for example, sponsorship, visibility, protection of time or status, and career-related opportunities; (2) the furnishing of support on a personal level through the provision of encouragement and counseling and the development of friendship; and (3) service as a role model for the mentee (Ensher, Heun, & Blanchard, 2003; Kram, 1985; Scandura, 1992). As a role model, the mentor may be acting as a "transfer agent of culture" in that he or she helps to shape values and serve as an example to mentees (Wilson & Elman, 1990). How these functions are carried out, the factors that may determine the success or failure of the mentoring relationship, and the models that may be used to effect these goals are the focus of the following discussion.

PHASES OF THE MENTORING RELATIONSHIP

Mentoring is not a static process. Rather, the functions implicit in mentoring and the nature and intensity of the mentoring relationship evolve and change over time. Various conceptualizations of this process have been advanced by a number of scholars. Despite the difference in terminology and the allocation of various functions to different phases, the conceptualization of the phases across scholars is similar in many aspects. Table 1.1 outlines the phases of the mentoring process as perceived by various researchers and the functions associated with each phase.

As can be seen, Kochan and Trimble (2000) are unique in their delineation of a "groundwork" phase prior to the selection of the mentor, during which time the mentee bears responsibility for a self-assessment of strengths, weaknesses, and goals. The initiation or preparation phase envisioned by Kram (1985) and Barker (2006) refers to the mutual selection of the mentor and mentee. In this conceptualization, the initiation phase would also encompass the identification of mentor and mentee responsibilities, a task that Zachery (2002) allocates to his second phase of negotiation and that Kochan and Trimble assign to their second phase, labeled warm-up. Kram (1985) and Barker's (2006) second phase of cultivation is similar to Zachery's (2002) third phase of enabling and Kochan and Trimble's third phase of working, a period of time during which learning is maximized and the mentoring relationship is at its most intense. Perhaps the greatest difference between the varied formulations of the mentoring relationship occurs toward its termination. Kram (1985), Barker (2006), and Kochan and Trimble (2000) conceive of a separation phase and an evolution of the mentoring relationship into one between colleagues, whereas Zachery (2002) seems to envision an actual termination of the relationship.

These varied conceptualizations share several common themes. First, the mentoring process moves through a number of developmental stages, during which the mentor fosters the increasing independence of his or her mentee and the mentee proceeds with increasing levels of self-sufficiency and self-direction. Second, and importantly, both the mentor and the mentee bear responsibility for the success of the relationship. Third, each of these stages encompasses specific tasks. These stages and their associated tasks are explored below. Further examples of these stages and the tasks associated with each can be found in the case studies provided by Horwitz and colleagues (Case Study 2; see Chapter 2) and Rice and Grusky (Case Study 5; see Chapter 5).

TABLE 1.1

Stages of the Mentoring Relationship and Their Associated Responsibilities

Author(s)	Phases of Mentoring Relationship	Mentor Tasks	Mentee Tasks	Shared Tasks	Mentee Skills Developed/Enhanced
Barker, 2006; Kram, 1985	Initiation: the mutual selection of the dyad (0–1 year)			Parties formulate expectations Relationship gains importance	
	Cultivation: the period of peak mentoring (2–5 years)		Gain sense of mastery and self-worth	Mismatches related to values, work style, or personality identified	
	Separation: termination of the mentoring relationship (after 2–5 years)	Mentor attempts to have mentee become more independent Mentor serves as a resource person	Mentee's autonomy and independence increase		Increased independence
	Redefinition: establishment of a peer relationship (several years after separation)	Provides occasional functions			Development of collegial relationships

(Continued)

5

TABLE 1.1 (*Continued*)
Stages of the Mentoring Relationship and Their Associated Responsibilities

Author(s)	Phases of Mentoring Relationship	Mentor Tasks	Mentee Tasks	Shared Tasks	Mentee Skills Developed/Enhanced
Fox, Rothrock, & Skelton, 1992	Recognition and development				
	Limited independence				Development of greater independence
	Termination and realignment				Ending relationships
Gefke, 1999	Phase 1			Get acquainted Build rapport	Communication
	Phase 2		Set goals Develop action plan	Contracting	Goal setting Negotiation Organization Personal responsibility Planning
	Phase 3		Implement plan	Assess program	Self-evaluation Reflection
	Phases 4–5		Reprioritize Develop additional goals	Evaluate success Reassess progress	Reflection
	Phase 6			Evaluation Separation	Transitioning relationships

Kochan & Trimble, 2000				
Groundwork		Mentee assessment of his/her strengths, weaknesses, and goals Identification of potential mentors		Personal responsibility Self-analysis Goal setting Networking Self-development
Warm-up: Establishment of relationship	Establish behavioral expectations Assist mentee to establish priorities	Identify priorities Clarify goals	Open communication Engage in active listening Develop schedule of meetings	Communication ability Develop appropriate level of assertiveness Priority setting Organization
Working: the height of the mentoring relationship	Assist mentee to develop relevant knowledge base Assist mentee in socialization into the profession and development of broader professional network	Develop knowledge base in field Continue to develop professional identity Develop broader professional network	Provide and receive constructive criticism Negotiate relationship boundaries (personal and professional)	Communication ability Reflection Collaboration Acceptance of feedback Negotiation
Long-term status: Nurturance of evolved relationship or termination			Discuss and process issues affecting relationship Nurture or discontinue relationship	Communication ability Adaptability

(Continued)

7

TABLE 1.1 (*Continued*)

Stages of the Mentoring Relationship and Their Associated Responsibilities

Author(s)	Phases of Mentoring Relationship	Mentor Tasks	Mentee Tasks	Shared Tasks	Mentee Skills Developed/Enhanced
Phillips, 1977	Mutual admiration				Initiating relationships
	Development				Developing relationships
	Disillusionment				
	Parting				Ending relationship
	Transformation				
Zachery, 2002	Preparation			Identify the match between the mentor and the mentee	
	Negotiation			Identify the responsibilities of the mentor and the mentee	Goal setting
				Define goals and what constitutes success	
	Enabling	Facilitate learning	Engage in learning		
	Closure and exit			Assess the learning situation	Communication
				Implement exit strategy	Transitioning relationships

BUILDING THE SUCCESSFUL MENTORING RELATIONSHIP

Laying the Groundwork

Mentor and Mentee Responsibilities and Preparation

Clearly, individuals must first be willing to enter into a relationship even before they begin to lay the groundwork for a specific relationship. Scholars have used social exchange theory (Thibaut & Kelley, 1959) to explain why individuals may be willing to enter into a mentoring relationship (Ensher, Thomas, & Murphy, 2001). Social exchange theory posits that individuals are willing to invest in a relationship and respond to that relationship based on their beliefs and perceptions of the costs and benefits associated with the relationship. One can conceive of this as essentially a cost-benefit analysis to help one decide whether to initiate, remain in, and/or terminate the relationship. The greater the benefits associated with the particular relationship, the more likely it will be initiated and maintained. Conversely, the greater the costs of establishing or continuing the relationship, the less likely individuals will be to enter into it or to continue with it (Sprecher, 1992). Clearly, however, the mentoring relationship can be marked by both positive and negative experiences and by both costs and benefits (Eby, Butts, Lockwood, & Simon, 2004). The importance of exchange theory is reflected in Rice's and Grusky's account of their joint mentoring experience (Case Study 5; see Chapter 5).

Empirical research with both mentors and mentees has linked several factors with the willingness to serve as a mentor. Individuals who have participated in a mentoring relationship in the past, either as a mentor or a mentee, appear to be more willing to accept the role of a mentor (Allen et al., 1997; Ragins & Cotton, 1993). Allen (2003) identified three primary incentives for individuals to agree to mentor others: for the purpose of self-enhancement, for the benefit of others, and for intrinsic satisfaction. A willingness to serve as a mentor has also been found to be associated with an internal locus of control, an upward striving (Allen et al., 1997), a sense of altruism (Allen, Poteet, & Burroughs, 1997), and organization-based self-esteem (Aryee, Chay, & Chew, 1996). Organizational factors may also play a critical role in individuals' willingness or lack thereof to serve as mentors; these are addressed in Chapter 5.

A willingness to serve as a mentor or to align oneself as a mentee is not, however, a sufficient foundation for a successful mentor–mentee relationship, the career development of the mentee, or the career validation of the mentor. As Kochan and Trimble (2000) suggest, the mentee must invest a significant amount of time preparing him- or herself for the responsibilities that attend the status of mentee. Similarly, prospective mentors must receive appropriate training that will help them work with their mentees in a manner that will be productive to each. Indeed, the adequate preparation of prospective mentors has been identified as a crucial prerequisite to the success of mentoring relationships (Dilbert & Goldenberg, 1995; Woodrow, 1994).

Kochan and Trimble (2000) recommend the use of various instruments to assist the mentee in his or her preparation for the mentoring relationship. The Thomas–Kilmann Conflict Mode Instrument (Thomas & Kilman, 1991), the Power Base Inventory (Thomas & Thomas, 1991), the Gregorc Style Delineator (Gregorc, 1985), and the Myers–Briggs Type Indicator (Myers & McCaulley, 1985) can be helpful in the identification of strengths, weaknesses, and manner of approaching situations. The results of these inventories can then provide a basis for the mentee's formulation of goals, which may, in turn, help the mentee to identify individuals who may be appropriate as mentors (Kochan & Trimble, 2000). Mentee preparation and evaluation are discussed more fully in Chapter 5.

Various approaches to mentor preparation have been suggested. These include the development of a comprehensive mentor training program (Wright-Harp & Cole, 2008), the establishment of a formal selection process for individuals to qualify for selection as a mentor (Miller, Devaney, Kelly, & Kuehn, 2008; Verdajo, 2002), and the requirement of a formal mentor–mentee contract that sets forth the mentor obligations in the relationship (Wright-Harp & Cole, 2008). Suggested learning strategies that can be used in a structured curriculum for mentor training include the use of written and audiovisual materials (Cotter et al., 2004), role-playing exercises (Miller et al., 2008), reflective exercises, and problem solving in small groups (Mills, Lennon, & Francis, 2006). Content areas to be addressed within a structured curriculum include the benefits of mentoring; the phases of the mentoring relationship; strategies to increase a mentee's competence, sense of self-esteem, and career opportunities; identification of and solutions to potential difficulties in the mentoring relationship; fostering institutional support for mentoring; integration and synthesis (Alleman et al., 1984); communication and behavioral styles (Mills et al., 2006); the identification and resolution of communication difficulties; and preexisting assumptions and expectations (Miller et al., 2008). Mentor training is discussed in greater detail in Chapter 5 in the context of the development and evaluation of mentoring programs.

The Selection Process: Matching Mentors and Mentees

Various elements have been identified for the development of a successful mentoring relationship. These include having an understanding of the nature of the relationship, monitoring the relationship as it progresses, having a realistic view of the relationship, exploring the compatibility of styles and objectives of the prospective mentor and mentee prior to entering into the relationship, and understanding and accepting the evolution of the relationship (Barker, 2006). Satisfaction with the mentoring relationship (Ensher & Murphy, 1997) and the type of mentoring support received (Ensher, Grant-Valone, & Marelich, 2002) appear to be greater when the mentor and mentee both perceive similarity in goals, attitudes, and beliefs.

Numerous studies have attempted to identify the personal attributes of mentors and mentees that may be critical to the success of a mentoring relationship. These are summarized in Table 1.2. Interestingly, many more studies have focused on the qualities of the mentor than on the characteristics of the mentee, despite the recognition that a mentoring relationship places responsibilities and demands on both the mentor and the mentee.

At first glance, it might appear that perfection in all aspects of one's personality and behavior is to be expected from mentors. Research suggests that such unrealistic expectations are more prevalent in the context of

TABLE 1.2

Summary of Needed Mentor and Mentee Qualities for Instrumental and Psychosocial Support in a Successful Mentoring Relationship

Mentor Qualities	Mentee Qualities	Qualities Needed by Both Mentor and Mentee
Ability to engage in active listening	Ability to analyze and synthesize material	Ability to communicate well
Accepting	Ability and willingness to reshape behavior	Ability to use feedback constructively
Caring	Belief in importance of interpersonal relationships	Self-awareness
Committed	Belief in importance of interpersonal relationships	
Competent	of interpersonal relationships	
Empathic	relationships	
Encouraging	Desire to learn	
Enthusiastic	High level of involvement in work	
Experienced	in work	
Expert in the field	Internal locus of control	
Friendly	Learning goal orientation	
Helpful		
Inspirational		
Intellectually stimulating		
Motivating		
Nonjudgmental		
Open minded		
Professional		
With a sense of altruism		
Sensitive to environment		
Sincere		
Supportive		

Compiled from Allen, 2003; Alred, Garvey, & Smith, 1998; Dancer, 2003; Darling, 1984; Freeman, 2004; Godshalk & Sosik, 2000, 2003; Hauer, Teherani, Dechet, & Aagaard, 2005; Kram, 1985; Larkin, 2003; Mills et al., 2006; Noe, 1988.

formal mentoring relationships, compared with those that are more informal (Murray, 1991; Ragins & Cotton, 1999; Zey, 1985); this is explored more fully in the section of this chapter focusing on models of mentoring. Scholars who view mentors and the mentoring process more realistically recognize the impossibility of fulfilling such expectations and that difficulties in the relationship may occur. Instead, they focus on the mutuality of learning that is inherent in the process and the humanness of that endeavor:

> Effective mentors are willing to confidently show their own challenges and frustrations. They act as facilitators of discovery, not teachers. Such leaders remove the masks of position as they demonstrate enthusiasm for learning. Great mentors guide the development of wisdom by working as hard to learn as they do to help another learn. (Bell, 1997, p. 15)

It is also important to note that the qualities associated with the successful provision of instrumental support to a mentee may differ from those that are required for the successful provision of psychosocial support. For example, Allen (2003) found from her survey study involving 253 individuals, 178 of whom had served at one time as a mentor, that the quality of helpfulness was associated with the successful provision of instrumental support; the quality of empathy, rather than helpfulness, was important for the provision of psychosocial support.

Perhaps one of the more critical mentee qualities that can contribute to the success of the mentoring relationship is that of *learning goal orientation*. This term refers to an individual's predisposition to seek out tasks that are challenging, to continue to strive even in difficult circumstances, and to treat failures as experiences that provide useful feedback (Button, Mahireu, & Zajak, 1996). The trait, which is considered to be relatively stable within an individual (Dweck, 1986), allows individuals to feel competent even with experiences of failure and to seek additional knowledge that will help them to further their careers (Godshalk & Sosik, 2003). In a study involving 245 adult students in a master of business administration program, including individuals employed in the health care industry, researchers found that mentees who shared high levels of learning goal orientation with their mentors reported higher levels of career satisfaction and managerial aspirations compared with mentees who shared low levels of learning goal orientation with their mentors (Godshalk & Sosik, 2003).

Phase 2, Cultivation and the Peaks and Pitfalls of Mentoring Relationships

Much has been written about the benefits to be obtained by the mentees of a successful mentoring relationship. A meta-analysis of studies relating to mentoring within an organizational setting concluded that there is a strong relationship between objective indicators of career success, for example, level of compensation and promotion, and career mentoring, that is, mentor sponsorship, coaching, and protection of the mentee, often made possible because of the more senior person's experience and position (Allen, Eby, Poteet, Lentz, & Lima, 2004; Kram, 1983). Career mentoring is to be distinguished, however, from job mentoring (Eby, 1997). Job mentoring tends to be organization specific and focused on job-related skill development within that organization, such as supporting the mentee's advancement, enhancing the mentee's visibility, and providing the mentee with advice about career opportunities potentially available within that organization. In contrast, career mentoring attempts to broaden the mentee's vision and experience beyond that of a particular organization. As an example, the mentor might promote the mentee's efforts both inside and outside of the organization, discuss alternative career options, and help the mentee to stay informed about current developments in his or her field (Eby, 1997).

The informational and instrumental social support provided through mentoring helps mentees to feel more confident in their career decisions and enhances their career-related efficacy. The psychosocial mentoring provided to a mentee through role modeling, acceptance, validation, counseling, and friendship appears to enhance the mentee's career satisfaction (Allen et al., 2004; Kram, 1983).

Social learning theory has been used in efforts to understand the relationship between mentoring and the mentee's career success. Social learning theory suggests that mentees learn by modeling their more senior mentors, who help the mentees learn the rules that govern appropriate behavior within a particular context (Bolton, 1980; Manz & Sims, 1981; Dreher & Ash, 1990; Zagumny, 1993).

Mentoring may also, however, offer benefits to the mentor. First, the mentor's career may be enhanced through the mentoring relationship (Zey, 1984). Mentors' visibility within their organization may be increased. Second, mentees may be a source of information for the mentor (Mullen, 1994; Zey, 1984), bringing fresh energy and a new perspective to the mentor's work (Kram, 1985; Levinson, Darrow, Klein, Levinson, & McKee, 1978). A mentoring relationship provides mentors with the opportunity to serve in an advisory role (Zey, 1984). Finally, the mentor may receive psychic rewards from the relationship (Zey, 1984) as the result of recognition from one's peers and superiors, a feeling of self-validation (Hunt & Michael, 1983), a sense of satisfaction at having helped others, and the development of close relationships (Allen et al., 1997).

Barriers, however, may stand in the way of forming any mentoring relationship and impede the development of a successful one. Medical students, for example, have identified their own career indecision, their inability to access non–university-based clinicians who might serve as mentors, faculty members' hectic schedules, and the lack of value placed on mentoring by medical school administrations as barriers to mentoring (Aagaard & Hauer, 2003). Research findings suggest that the students' perceptions may be accurate, at least to some degree. Researchers conducting an interview study with 27 mentor-participants, including individuals in the health care field, reported that the primary barrier to individuals' assumption of mentor responsibilities was the time required by such a responsibility (Allen et al., 1997).

Even after the establishment of a mentoring relationship, negative experiences may dissuade the mentor and/or the mentee from pursuing or continuing the relationship. A mismatch between the values, personalities, or workstyles of the mentor and mentee may occur during any phase of the mentoring relationship. This mismatch may lead to disagreements and unpleasantness (Kram, 1985), resulting in early termination of the mentoring relationship. Mentors may also negatively affect the mentoring relationship through self-absorption or inattention to the career needs of the mentee (Eby, McManus, Simon, & Russell, 2000). As the mentee gains increasing independence and autonomy, the mentor may become threatened and, as a result, become tyrannical, sabotage the mentee's work (Levinson et al., 1978), exploit the mentee (Tobin, 2004), take credit for the mentee's work (Beech & Brockbank, 1999; Eby et al., 2000; Tobin, 2004), prevent the mentee's advancement (Ragins & Scandura, 1997), or exclude the mentee from participation (Eby et al., 2000). Eby and Allen (2002) have grouped these behaviors into five broader metathemes: mismatch within the mentor–mentee dyad, mentor distancing behavior, mentor manipulative behavior, lack of mentor expertise, and general dysfunctionality of the mentor. In the most egregious situations, the mentor may engage in sexual harassment of the mentee (Hurley & Fagenson-Eland, 1996; Scandura, 1998). Such negative experiences with a mentor have been associated with mentee depression and job withdrawal (Eby et al., 2004).

Negative experiences of mentees with their mentors appear to be so common that several scholars developed a classification scheme for what has been called "toxic mentors" (Darling, 1985; Stone, 2005, cited as personal communication in Barker, 2006, p. 58). "Avoiders" rarely make themselves available to provide advice or guidance, despite their assertion that they are accessible. "Dumpers" believe that the mentee is totally responsible for the acquisition of knowledge and the development of necessary skills and that the mentor is not responsible in any way to facilitate this process. Indeed, the maxim of such mentors is "sink or swim." *Blockers* impede the mentee's success by micromanaging his or her work or by withholding information that is critical to the work's success. "Destroyers" undermine and sabotage their mentees, believing that constant criticism is the best preparation for their entry into their profession. "Smotherers" believe that any idea of the mentee is their own idea and any product of the mentee is similarly their own (Stone, 2005, cited as personal communication in Barker, 2006, p. 58).

Mentee behaviors may also give rise to difficulties within the mentoring relationship as well. Some mentees may align themselves with the mentor in the belief that they will be able to gain power; they may make unauthorized statements in the name of the mentor, creating the impression that they hold more power and knowledge than they actually do (Stone, 2005, cited as personal communication in Barker, 2006, p. 59). Mentees may also become jealous or resentful of their mentor's position and use innuendo, compromise collaborations or negotiations, or "backstab" their mentor in an attempt to undermine the mentor (Barker, 2006; Halatin & Knotts, 1982; Ragins & Scandura, 1994). Mentees with multiple mentors may play mentors off against each other rather than assuming responsibility for their own behaviors and decisions (Nolinske, 1995).

Various approaches have been suggested to address negative experiences that may arise during a mentoring relationship. The problem must be identified clearly. Once the problem has been defined, the nature of the problem and its development can be monitored by the mentor and the mentee through the use of their own journals. Each should attempt to keep an open line of communication, develop an external source of support, practice encounters before they occur, use a facilitator during termination discussions, and document the proceedings (Barker, 2006).

This writer also suggests that a facilitator be brought into any discussions that may be difficult or problematic, not only those involving the possibility of termination. In many instances, a skilled third party may perceive the difficulties in the communication between the mentor and mentee and help to "translate" what is being said so that each can better hear the other. In some situations, particularly those that are characterized by hostility between the parties, it may be important to have a third party present who can record the meeting and/or verify what was said during the meeting in the event that issues are raised later with respect to what may have transpired.

Phase 3, Separation

Separation may occur in the natural course of the mentoring relationship, or it may occur quite unexpectedly. A planned separation may come about following the completion of the mentee's program, such as following the conclusion of a postdoctoral fellow's training; due to the mentor's or mentee's departure for another institution; or the mentor's retirement (Bhagia & Tinsley, 2000). A sudden or unexpected separation may occur because of the unexpected illness or death of the mentor or the mentee.

Mentee responses to the separation may vary widely. In situations in which the separation has been planned, the mentor and mentee can share their feelings about the upcoming changes and plan for future contact.

There is often sufficient time to grieve the ending of the relationship as it has been known and to look forward with excitement to its next phase.

An unexpected separation due to the death of the mentor or mentee may provoke widely differing emotions including grief, anger, regret, guilt, and a sense of loss. In situations in which the mentor and mentee shared a close relationship, the remaining dyadic member may feel as though he or she has lost a close friend or family member (Bhagia & Tinsley, 2000). A variety of strategies may be helpful to overcome the grief, such as interacting with mutual colleagues and friends, confiding in friends, and honoring one's feelings of loss.

Phase 4, Redefinition

The redefinition phase occurs several years after separation. This phase is characterized by a movement in the relationship to encompass more personal issues (cf. Kochan & Trimble, 2000). The mentor and the mentee view each other as colleagues; they may share their personal and professional frustrations and aspirations and plan collaborations.

MODELS OF MENTORING

The Classic Mentoring Model

Much, if not most, of the research that has been conducted on the phases or stages of mentoring has focused on the dyadic model, which is best known as the classic or traditional model of mentoring. The dyadic mentoring relationship may be formal or informal.

Formal mentoring is planned and defined within the specific setting in which it occurs (Golian & Galbraith, 1996). Researchers conducting a study of perceived program characteristics, program effectiveness, satisfaction with mentors, and job attitudes related to formal mentoring involving 104 mentees in the fields of social work, engineering, and journalism found that meeting frequency was related to perceived program effectiveness (Ragins, Cotton, & Miller, 2000). Additionally, having a mentor from a different department was associated with increased organizational commitment, fewer intentions to quit, and greater satisfaction with the mentor. However, other studies have found that mentees whose supervisors served as mentors for them are more comfortable communicating with their mentors than were mentees whose mentors are more distanced in the organization (Burle, McKenna, & McKeen, 1991), that mentor-supervisors have greater knowledge of their mentees' needs and are often required by their organization to be attentive to their mentees' needs (Ragins & McFarlin,

1990), and that mentor-supervisors provide more career guidance and psychosocial support to their mentees than do non–supervisor-mentors (Fagenson-Eland, Marks, & Amendola, 1997; Ragins & McFarlin, 1990).

Variations of formal mentoring include the "trans" and the "cis" designs (Kahn & Greenblatt, 2009). The "trans" model involves pairing a mentee with a mentor who works outside of the mentee's area of focus. As an example, a mentee engaged in clinical research might be paired with a senior researcher who is a basic scientist. The "trans" design offers several advantages, including a reduced likelihood of duplicating mentoring efforts from the mentee's own department, facilitating the mentee's identification of new colleagues, promoting the mentee's development of a larger professional network, and fostering multidisciplinary, multidepartmental collaborations (Brownson, Samet, & Thacker, 2002; Chapman, Sellaeg, Levy-Milne, & Barr, 2007). The "trans" design has been used successfully in a mentoring program for early career scientists in HIV research at the University of California, San Francisco (Kahn & Greenblatt, 2009).

In comparison to the "trans" design, the "cis" design matches a mentee with a mentor from the same discipline (Kahn & Greenblatt, 2009). As an example, a mentee conducting behavioral research would be matched with a mentor in the same fields. This approach may be more susceptible to the potential difficulties discussed earlier in this chapter.

In contrast to formal mentoring, informal mentoring is

> a relationship that occurs that is unplanned, and, in most cases, not expected. A certain "chemistry" emerges drawing two individuals together for the purpose of professional, personal, and psychological growth and development. Informal mentoring seems to be a qualitative experience that has great meaning for the parties involved. (Golian & Galbraith, 1996, p. 102)

The success of informal mentoring relationships has been attributed to the interpersonal dynamics of these relationships, such as reciprocal liking and attraction (Kram, 1985; Ragins & Cotton, 1999).

Although research suggests that formal mentoring is better than no mentoring, it is less effective than informal mentoring (Chao, Walz, & Gardner, 1992) and may not offer any career advantage over individuals who are not mentored at all (Ragins & Cotton, 1999). This may be due to the nature of the interpersonal processes that underlie more informal mentoring. Scholars have speculated that because formal mentoring programs often involve the matching of the mentor and mentee by a third party, there is a decreased likelihood that the pair will be able to work together amicably or will like each other (Ragins & Cotton, 1999). (Strategies for improved mentor–mentee matching are addressed in Chapter 5.) Additionally, individuals who believe that their participation in such a program is mandated may be less inclined to devote adequate time and energy to the relationship; mentors may neglect the mentee, or mentees may resist learning from the mentor (Eby & McManus, 2004; Eby et al., 2000; Kram & Hall, 1996). Mentor–mentee communication appears to be less informal, compared with informal mentoring relationships (Fagenson-Eland et al., 1997). Researchers have found that distancing behavior and a lack of mentor expertise more frequently occur in the context for formal, rather than informal, mentoring (Eby et al., 2004).

Accordingly, the incorporation of various elements into formal mentoring programs so as to mimic the processes of informal mentoring programs and thereby increase their effectiveness has been suggested (Greenhaus, Callanan, & Godshalk, 2000; Wanberg, Welsh, & Hezlett, 2003). These strategies include allowing individuals to feel both as if they have input into the mentor–mentee matching process and that the process is voluntary; increasing opportunities for interaction between the mentor and mentee; and considering rank and departmental differences in matching mentees and mentors, in an effort to facilitate and maximize learning and the development of emotional ties (Greenhaus et al., 2000). Indeed, research findings indicate a positive association between perceived input into the matching process and mentor and mentee perceptions of the quality of the mentoring relationship (Allen, Eby, & Lentz, 2006).

Formal mentoring relationships may also be plagued by more negative experiences than are informal ones. Formal mentoring relationships tend to be more highly visible. They may be promoted, endorsed, and publicized by the entity that establishes them; their high profile may inadvertently create unrealistic expectations in the minds of the mentees, leading to dissatisfaction and disappointment. Such circumstances may lead the mentee to believe that he or she is unable to terminate a mentoring relationship that is not working well (Eby & Allen, 2002).

The classic model of mentoring, whether informal or formal, has been criticized by various feminist scholars. They have argued that the traditional dyadic model of mentoring is essentially geared to grooming or growing others who are clones of their mentors and will replicate the existing culture, a scenario that leaves few possibilities for women's growth or upward movement in the field (Blackburn, Chapman, & Cameron, 1981; Swoboda & Millar, 1986). It has been suggested that reliance on a single mentor is especially unrealistic for women entering the sciences and that nontraditional models of mentoring, such as networking and having multiple mentors, should be seriously considered (Nolinske, 1995; Swoboda & Millar, 1986). The networking model is less intense than the traditional dyadic model of mentoring, provides the mentee with a broader range of perspectives, and avoids the difficulties associated with overdependence on one mentor and limitations that develop from exposure to only one perspective. However, the mentee must then assume greater responsibility for his or her own professional growth and development (Nolinske, 1995;

Swoboda & Millar, 1986). (The networking model is described in greater depth in a later section.) Mentoring issues relevant to women are explored in greater detail in Chapter 4, focusing on diversity.

The Preceptorship Model

The preceptorship model is similar to the classic model of mentoring in that it is a dyadic relationship between an individual who is more experienced and one who is less experienced in the relevant field. In this model, the mentor is responsible for creating opportunities for the mentee to practice the relevant skills. This model may be implemented in an attempt to reduce staff turnover, to recognize the experts in the organization, and to guide recent entrants to the profession (Greene & Puetzer, 2002). As an example, one entity commenced a mentoring program for nurses using this model to reduce the enormous frequent staff turnover (Greene & Puetzer, 2002).

The MCP (Medical College of Pennsylvania) Hahnemann University National Center of Leadership in Academic Medicine was particularly innovative in its reliance on a preceptorship model. Partly in response to major organizational changes, the Center established a two-tier system of mentoring (Benson, Morahan, Sachdeva, & Richman, 2002). The first tier, consisting of a 1-year precepting program, was designed to orient new faculty to the School of Medicine and MCP Hahnemann University, lessen the anxiety that new faculty may experience, increase faculty members' productivity in a shortened time, and increase their potential to succeed. The second tier of the program, which reflected a more classic model of mentoring, was for a longer term and required that the mentor and mentee complete a formal agreement and an annual evaluation and meet on a regular basis. The adoption of this two-tier approach was found to facilitate recruitment of senior-level faculty as mentors, many of whom had limited time available due to the reorganization; with this shortened first tier commitment, they could limit the time commitment required. The program also seemed to encourage retention of minority faculty.

As the mentee becomes more experienced under the guidance of the mentor, he or she develops increasing confidence and self-efficacy. It appears that mentees participating in preceptorship mentoring relationships achieve greater benefits if they are able to select their mentor rather than having him or her assigned to them (Hayes, 1998).

The Shadowing Model

Scholars appear to differ on whether shadowing actually constitutes a model of mentoring or instead represents one component of an adequate mentoring relationship, but is not a model in and of itself. Shadowing allows less experienced professionals to observe those who are more experienced and to learn through this observation. As an example, student nurses have been paired with experienced nurses to participate in such activities as the negotiation of conflicts, the development of health policy, the assessment of medical compliance, and the creation of patient education protocols (Grossman, 2005). An evaluation of the program found that students who had participated had increased their leadership scores as measured by a standardized instrument (Grossman & Valiga, 2005).

The Peer or Co-Mentoring Model

Unlike the classical model of mentoring, in which the mentor generally possesses greater expertise, power, and position than his or her mentee, the co-mentoring model involves a relationship by parties who serve as mentors to each other; their relationship is characterized by flexibility of role and power between the parties (Norell & Ingoldsby, 1991). The degree of power and the role assumed by either individual in the co-mentoring relationship are a direct function of the specific project at hand and the skills, knowledge, and talents that each individual brings to that project. Essentially, each individual in the relationship takes his or her turn as counselor, sponsor, adviser, and teacher.

A co-mentor should not be thought of as equivalent to a co-worker relationship, although a co-mentor may be a co-worker. Unlike a relationship with a co-worker, a co-mentoring relationship is characterized by intentionality and an active search for strategies that can be used for mutual support and career development (Norell & Ingoldsby, 1991). It has been suggested that, in a co-mentoring relationship, each of the partners is responsible for the other's learning (Beattie & McDougall, 1994). As such, peer mentoring is equivalent to what has been termed *peer learning partnerships* (Eisen, 2001). These are "voluntary, reciprocal helping relationships between individuals of comparable status, who share a common or closely related learning/development objective" (Eisen, 2000, p. 5). This type of mentoring helps individuals to develop a feeling of being equal to others in the field (Blackwell, 1996) and also helps to establish a culture of learning (Beattie & McDougall, 1994). This model may be preferable to the classical model for the mentoring of professionals in the early stages of their careers because it recognizes and builds upon the individual's existing expertise (Eisen, 2001).

Examples of a peer mentoring model include the mentoring program available to nursing students through the National Student Nurses Association (http://www.nsna.org) by networking with other students and nurses throughout the country and the Teaching Partners Program (TPP) in Connecticut. The TPP seeks to enhance its participants' teaching practices through observation of and surveys conducted with the students of the participating teacher's co-mentor; regular feedback between the partners in the co-mentoring dyad to review findings and explore alternative approaches to learning and teaching; and the preparation by each co-mentor of reflective reports detailing his or her experiences (Eisen, 2001). The co-mentoring occurs over the course of two consecutive semesters. Each participant is provided with a stipend to offset the intensive time commitment required for his or her participation. A group peer, collaborative mentoring model premised on the principles of adult education has also been used successfully with junior faculty in academic medicine (Pololi & Knight, 2005; Pololi, Knight, Dennis, & Frankel, 2002). This program is discussed in greater detail in Chapter 2.

The Interagency Model

One of the more recently proposed innovations to mentor models is that of the interagency model. This model has been used to support management development and build management capacity in responding more effectively to structural and policy changes within the health care sector (Hafford-Letchfield & Chick, 2006). One of the primary benefits derived from this approach is the development of "transcendent" managers who are able to navigate organizational barriers (Hafford-Letchfield & Chick, 2006, p. 17).

A steering committee composed of representatives from the various participating agencies bears responsibility for matching mentors and mentees from different professional backgrounds and different agencies. These differences permit the cross-fertilization of ideas and perspectives while simultaneously laying a foundation for enhanced interagency cooperation and collaboration. A safe environment is created in which individuals are able to examine and to reflect critically on their beliefs and values that they may have taken for granted in their own organizational environments.

The Networking Model

As indicated above, the networking model requires that the mentee assume the initiative to identify individuals, groups, and organizations that can provide him or her with mentoring experiences (Packard, 2003). This allows the individual to develop a constellation of mentors that will provide him or her with diverse perspectives; indeed, a mentor in such an arrangement may be able to address only one particular aspect of the mentee's professional development. Because there are multiple relationships that are relatively less intense than that developed in a traditional mentoring model, there is a reduced likelihood of incompatibility between the mentor and the mentee (Swoboda & Millar, 1986).

The Multiple Mentoring Model

There has been an increased recognition in recent years that more than one mentor may be necessary to promote the successful career development of individuals in the health sciences. Not infrequently, a potential mentor may possess either expertise in the content area of the mentee's proposed work or the professional connections that are necessary to build a professional network but not both. Reliance on a multiple mentor model offers an opportunity for more than one mentor, each with a specific set of skills and a different perspective that offer potential benefit for the mentee's career trajectory. This model is distinguishable from the networking model by its inclusion of fewer mentors and the greater intensity of the relationship that exists between the mentee and his or her mentors.

De Janasz, Sullivan, Whiting, and Biech (2003) have suggested that an intelligent career encompasses three competencies: knowing why, or the fit between one's own identity and one's career choice; knowing how, referring to the skills and knowledge needed to carry out one's profession; and knowing whom, that is, the relationships that comprise an individual's network. They assert that different mentors are needed to assist individuals in their development of these three competencies; these mentors together constitute "an intelligent mentor network" (de Janasz et al., 2003, p. 84). They identified five steps as a prerequisite to the establishment of an intelligent network: (1) the investment by the mentee of the time and energy necessary to establish and maintain a network of developmental relationships (becoming the perfect protégé); (2) the mentee's integration of his or her social life with work contacts and friendships ("a 360-degree" network); (3) the mentee's commitment to assessing, constructing, and adjusting his or her mentor network; (4) the mentee's development of diverse, synergistic connections that extend beyond organization or institutional boundaries; and (5) the mentee's recognition that change is inevitable and that everything—whether it is good, bad, or indifferent—comes to an end (de Janasz et al., 2003, pp. 84–87). One example of a multiple mentoring model is that provided by Horwitz and colleagues in Case Study 2.

Wright-Harp and Cole (2008) have recommended reliance on a five-tier mentoring model to enhance the success of graduate students in human communication sciences and disorders. However, this model may be adapted for graduate students across health-related disciplines. The five-tier model consists of five mentors: an academic mentor, a clinical mentor, a research mentor, a peer mentor, and a career/professional development mentor. The academic mentor would very often be the same individual as the mentee's academic adviser, helping the mentee to select appropriate courses and facilitating the mentee's introduction to other faculty and students in the field. The clinical mentor is relevant only for health-related fields that involve practical training or a practicum, such as nursing, social work, clinical psychology, physical therapy, and so on. Similarly, the research mentor is relevant only for those who are required to conduct research as part of their program. The peer mentor is an individual in the same academic field as the mentee but with at least slightly more senior status in the program. The career/professional development mentor is senior in his or her field, with a highly developed professional network that is potentially accessible to the mentee.

The multiple mentoring model can also assume the form of a team that includes both more senior members and members at the same level of their careers as the mentee (Eby, 1997). Team members can provide technical knowledge, set standards, provide performance monitoring and feedback (Hackman, 1992), and lobby for additional resources (Ancona & Caldwell, 1992).

The multiple mentoring model offers several advantages. Because the involvement between the mentor and mentee is less intense than it might be in a classic model, the mentor can potentially mentor a greater number of individuals simultaneously. The mentee will spend less time searching for the perfect mentor who can meet all of his or her needs. Additionally, an individual who has multiple mentors will be less impacted by a mentor who is dysfunctional or unavailable (de Janasz et al., 2003). For example, a study conducted with 1,432 faculty members at the University of Pennsylvania School of Medicine found that assistant professors who had two or more mentors were more likely to receive different forms of mentoring, different kinds of advice and different kinds of opportunities, and to report higher job satisfaction (Wasserstein, Quistberg, & Shea, 2007).

However, there are potential disadvantages of this model as well. Because there are multiple mentors, it is crucial that the mentors communicate with each other and coordinate their efforts. An irresponsible mentee can more easily avoid doing what is necessary because of the lesser degree of involvement of the mentors.

Mentoring Partnerships

Mentoring partnerships have become increasingly common in the academic setting as a mechanism for training individuals in the health professions. This arrangement consists of the pairing of a student, such as a nursing or medical school student, with a patient and a more experienced practitioner. This model provides the student with hands-on experience, the patient with additional medical attention, and the mentor with assistance in caring for the patient (McCadden, 2003).

Distance and e-Mentoring

Distance mentoring and e-mentoring are increasingly relied upon as models for mentoring. The recent increased utilization of these models is attributable to various factors including the lack of adequate expertise in a particular specialization in a particular geographic area, relative geographic isolation, time constraints, and a desire to promote "cross-fertilization" among geographically distant and diverse individuals (Miller et al., 2008; Paterson, McColl, & Paterson, 2004; Stewart & Carpenter, 2009). e-Mentoring has been found to be particularly useful in the provision of mentoring to health care professionals who practice in underserved rural and urban areas (Rockman, Salach, Gotlib, Cord, & Turner, 2004; Stewart & Carpenter, 2009). Additionally, distance and e-mentoring can be used in conjunction with other models of mentoring, such as the multiple mentor model and the network model.

Components of distance and e-mentoring programs may include regular e-mail correspondence, videoconferences, faxes, and iChat sessions (Stewart & Carpenter, 2009). These sessions may be supplemented with telephone calls and face-to-face interactions. Depending on the specific health discipline and the nature of the training, the various sessions may focus on caseload management, clinical issues, the identification of needed resources (Stewart & Carpenter, 2009), and the roles and values of the specific profession (Cascio & Gasker, 2001). Mentors may provide emotional support and validate mentees' experiences (Cascio & Gasker, 2001). Maintaining the confidentiality of transmitted data and the privacy of patients or research participants whose issues are discussed in the context of mentoring sessions may present challenges. It is therefore critical that mechanisms be established to handle issues of confidentiality and privacy before an e-mentoring program is actually begun (Ensher et al., 2003).

E-mentoring and distance mentoring offer many advantages. First, programs' use of a common discussion board permits both the mentor and the mentee to remain connected with multiple mentees and mentors (Miller et al., 2008). Second, individuals who may feel overburdened with time commitments and are consequently unable to provide face-to-face mentoring may be willing to serve as mentors if they are able to provide the necessary information and support while sitting in their offices or homes (Kalisch, Falzette, & Cooke, 2005). Third, the use of online mentoring allows mentors and mentees to use a variety of modalities for learning, teaching, and communicating, such as multimedia tutorials, videos, and so on (Ensher et al., 2003). Fourth, online mentoring may reduce any costs associated with mentoring. Fifth, online mentoring tends to equalize the status between the mentors and the mentees because individuals cannot see the superficial characteristics of the individuals with whom they are communicating (Ensher et al., 2003). Positive outcomes of e-mentoring programs for mentees include improved clinical reasoning, increased confidence and knowledge, informal sharing, increased collaboration, and the availability of support (Stewart & Carpenter, 2009).

One example of successful online/e-mentoring is that of MentorNet. This is a year-long program that matches undergraduate and graduate women with industry professionals in math, science, and engineering in an attempt to increase women's representation in these fields. The program was initiated in 1998 with funding from AT & T and Intel foundations. The program, which has matched more than 19,000 mentor–mentee pairs, has been found to increase participating mentees' self-confidence that they will succeed in their chosen field (MentorNet, 2007).

However, there are also barriers and drawbacks to an e-mentoring approach. e-Mentoring often uses e-mail as the primary mode of communication. Lack of access to a computer, unfamiliarity with e-mail, lack of computer skills (Rockman et al., 2004), or discomfort with writing (Ensher et al., 2003) may hinder mentor or mentee participation. Mentors' lack of response or delayed response may lead mentees to feel abandoned or disconnected (Miller et al., 2008; cf. Rideout, 2006). Miscommunications may be more likely to occur because of misinterpretations. It is more difficult to decipher tone in the context of e-mails than in face-to-face interactions, and a communication that may seem humorous to one individual may be emotionally charged to another. Individuals may erroneously believe that what they are writing electronically is private and may later be shocked to learn that the content of their writing is accessible to others or that it may become evidence in a lawsuit. Online relationships may develop more slowly than they would if they were face-to-face (Ensher et al., 2003). Computer malfunctions may also present frustrations and challenges.

Multilevel Mentoring

More recently, multilevel mentoring has been encouraged as a strategy to orient new faculty to academic medicine and to nurture their professional development (Lewellen-Williams et al., 2006). However, it is potentially relevant for mentoring in many health professions.

The multilevel Peer-Onsite-Distance (POD) model provides the mentee with peer, onsite, and distance mentors who focus on assisting the mentee to develop identified content and interaction skills. The peer mentors help to socialize the mentees to the academic environment and provide collegial support. The onsite mentors consist of senior faculty who provide the mentee with guidance and advice and fulfill coaching and advocacy functions. The distance mentors, who serve for a period of 1 year only, furnish the mentees with information relevant to their careers. This model has been used successfully with underrepresented minority faculty at the College of Medicine at the University of Arkansas for Medical Sciences (Lewellen-Williams et al., 2006).

SUMMARY

A mentoring relationship may assume any number of forms, ranging from the traditional dyadic model of mentoring to the more recently developed model of e-mentoring. Regardless of the specific model used, mentoring should provide the mentee with a supportive environment in which he or she can refine the content knowledge required for success in the relevant field, establish a network of professional relationships, and develop greater independence and self-efficacy as a health professional. A successful mentoring relationship may also address the needs of the mentor(s), which may include assistance with his or her research, the sharing of insights, and recognition by colleagues and/or the relevant institution for the mentoring effort. As with any relationship, mentoring relationships may encounter difficulties and will pass through various phases as the individuals in the relationship grow and change and as the relationship progresses. As illustrated in Case Study 1 by O'Shea and Lloyd, a successful mentoring relationship requires care, attention, and negotiation.

REFERENCES

Aagaard, E. M., & Hauer, K. E. (2003). A cross-sectional descriptive study of mentoring relationships formed by medical students. *Journal of General Internal Medicine, 18,* 298–302.

Alleman, E., Cochran, J., Doverspike, J., & Newman, I. (1984). Enriching mentoring relationship. *Personnel and Guidance Journal, 62,* 329–332.

Allen, T. D. (2003). Mentoring others: A dispositional and motivational approach. *Journal of Vocational Behavior, 62,* 134–154.

Allen, T. D., Eby, L. T., & Lentz, E. (2006). Mentorship behaviors and mentorship quality associated with formal mentoring programs: Closing the gap between research and practice. *Journal of Applied Psychology, 91*(3), 567–578.

Allen, T. D., Eby, L. T., Poteet, M. L., Lentz, E., & Lima, L. (2004). Career benefits associated with mentoring for protégés: A meta-analysis. *Journal of Applied Psychology, 89*(1), 127–136.

Allen, T. D., Poteet, M. L., & Burroughs, S. M. (1997). The mentor's perspective: A qualitative inquiry and future research agenda. *Journal of Vocational Behavior, 51,* 70–89.

Allen, T. D., Poteet, M. L., Russell, J. E. A., & Dobbins, G. H. (1997). A field study of factors related to supervisors' willingness to mentor others. *Journal of Vocational Behavior, 50,* 1–22.

Alred, G., Garvey, B., & Smith, R. (1998). *The mentoring pocket-book.* Alresford, UK: Alresford Press.

American Speech-Language Hearing Association. (2007). *ASHA 2006 member counts.* Retrieved October 29, 2010 from http://www.asha.org/about/membership-certification/member-data/member-counts.htm

Ancona, D. G., & Caldwell, D. F. (1992). Bridging the boundary: External activity and performance in organizational teams. *Administrative Science Quarterly, 37,* 634–665.

Anderson, E. M., & Shannon, A. L. (1988). Toward a conceptualization of mentoring. *Journal of Teacher Education, 39,* 38–42.

Aryee, S., Chay, Y. W., & Chew, J. (1996). The motivation to mentor among managerial employees. *Group & Organization Management, 21,* 261–277.

Barker, E. R. (2006). Mentoring—A complex relationship. *Journal of the American Academy of Nurse Practitioners, 18*(2), 56–61.

Barondess, J. A. (1995). President's address: A brief history of mentoring. *Transactions of the American Clinical and Climatological Association, 106,* 1–24.

Beattie, R. S., & McDougall, M. F. (1994). *Peer mentoring: A development strategy for the 1990s and beyond.* Paper for the European Mentoring Centre, Sheffield University. Cited in Wood, M. (1997). Mentoring in further and higher education: Learning from the literature. *Education + Training, 39*(9), 333–343.

Beech, N., & Brockbank, A. (1999). Power/knowledge and psychosocial dynamics in mentoring. *Management Learning, 30*(1), 7–25.

Bell, C. R. (1997). Intellectual capital. *Executive Excellence, 14,* 15–16.

Benson, C. A., Morahan, P. S., Sachdeva, A. K., & Richman, R. C. (2002). Effective faculty preceptoring and mentoring during reorganization of an academic medical center. *Medical Teacher, 24*(5), 550–557.

Bhagia, J., & Tinsley, J. A. (2000). The mentoring partnership. *Mayo Clinic Proceedings, 75*(5), 535–537.

Blackburn, R. T., Chapman, D., & Cameron, S. M. (1981). "Cloning" in academe: Mentorship and academic careers. *Research in Higher Education, 15,* 315–327.

Blackwell, J. E. (1989). Mentoring: An action strategy for increasing minority faculty. *Academe, 75,* 8–14.

Blackwell, R. (1996). In pursuit of the "feel equal" factor. *People Management, 2*(12), 36.

Bolton, E. B. (1980). A conceptual analysis of the mentor relationship in career development of women. *Adult Education, 30,* 195–207.

Brownson, R. C., Samet, J. M., & Thacker, S. B. (2002). Commentary: What contributes to a successful career in epidemiology in the United States? *American Journal of Epidemiology, 156,* 60–67.

Burle, R., McKenna, C., & McKeen, C. (1991). How do mentorships differ from typical supervisory relationships? *Psychological Reports, 68,* 459–466.

Burrell, B., Wood, S. J., Pikes, T., & Holliday, C. (2001). Student mentors and protégés learning together. *Teaching Exceptional Children, 3*(3), 24–29.

Button, S. B., Mathieu, J. E., & Zajac, D. M. (1996). Goal orientation in organizational research: A conceptual and empirical foundation. *Organizational Behavior and Human Decision Processes, 67*(1), 26–48.

Cascio, T., & Gasker, J. (2001). Everyone has a shining side: Computer-mediated mentoring in social work education. *Journal of Social Work Education, 37*(2), 283–293.

Chapman, G. E., Sellaeg, K., Levy-Milne, B., & Barr, S. L. (2007). Toward increased capacity for practice-based research among health professionals: Implementing a multisite qualitative research project with dietitians. *Qualitative Health Research, 17*, 902–907.

Chao, G. T., Walz, P., & Gardner, P. D. (1992). Formal and informal mentorships: A comparison of mentoring functions and contrast with nonmentored counterparts. *Personnel Psychology, 45*(3), 619–636.

Cotter, J. J., Coogle, C. L., Parham, I. A., Head, C., Fulton, L., Watson, K., et al. (2004). Designing a multi-disciplinary geriatrics health professional mentoring program. *Educational Gerontology, 30*, 107–117.

Dancer, J. M. (2003). Mentoring in healthcare: Theory in search of practice? *Clinician in Management, 12*, 21–31.

Darling, L. A. (1984). What do nurses want in a mentor? *The Journal of Nursing Administration, 14*, 42–44.

Darling, L. W. (1985). What to do about toxic mentors. *The Journal of Nursing Administration, 15*, 43–44.

de Janasz, S. C., Sullivan, S. E., Whiting, V., & Biech, E. (2003). Mentor networks and career success: Lessons for turbulent times. *The Academy of Management Executive, 17*(4), 78–93.

Dilbert, C., & Goldenberg, D. (1995). Preceptors' perceptions of benefits, rewards, supports, and commitment to the preceptor role. *Journal of Advanced Nursing, 21*, 1144–1151.

Dreher, G. F., & Ash, R. A. (1990). A comparative study of mentoring among men and women in managerial, professional, and technical positions. *Journal of Applied Psychology, 75*, 539–546.

Eby, L., Butts, M., Lockwood, A., & Simon, S. A. (2004). Protégés negative mentoring experiences: Construct development and nosological validation. *Personnel Psychology, 57*, 411–447.

Eby, L. T. (1997). Alternative forms of mentoring in changing organizational environments: A conceptual extension of the mentoring literature. *Journal of Vocational Behavior, 51*, 125–144.

Eby, L. T., & Allen, T. D. (2002). Further investigation of protégés negative mentoring experiences. *Group & Organization Management, 27*(4), 456–479.

Eby, L. T., & McManus, S. E. (2004). The protégé's role in negative mentoring experiences. *Journal of Vocational Behavior, 65*, 255–275.

Eby, L. T., McManus, S. E., Simon, S. A., & Russell, J. E. A. (2000). The protégé's perspective regarding negative mentoring experiences: The development of a taxonomy. *Journal of Vocational Behavior, 57*, 1–21.

Eisen, M.-J. (2000). Peer learning partnerships: Promoting reflective practice through reciprocal learning. *Inquiry: Critical Thinking Across the Disciplines, 19*(3), 5–19.

Eisen, M.-J. (2001). Peer-based professional development viewed through the lens of transformative learning. *Holistic Nurse Practitioner, 16*(1), 30–42.

Ensher, E. A., Grant-Valone, E., & Marelich, W. D. (2002). Effects of perceived attitudinal and demographic similarity on protégés support and satisfaction gained from their mentoring relationships. *Journal of Applied Social Psychology, 32*, 1–26.

Ensher, E. A., Heun, C., & Blanchard, A. (2003). Online mentoring and computer-mediated communication: New directions on research. *Journal of Vocational Behavior, 63*, 264–288.

Ensher, E. A., & Murphy, S. E. (1997). Effects of race, gender, perceived similarity, and contact on mentor relationships. *Journal of Vocational Behavior, 50*, 460–481.

Ensher, E. A., Thomas, C., & Murphy, S. E. (2001). Comparison of traditional, step-ahead, and peer mentoring on protégés' support, satisfaction, and perception of career success: A social exchange perspective. *Journal of Business and Psychology, 15*(3), 419–438.

Fagenson-Eland, E. A., Marks, M. A., & Amendola, K. L. (1997). Perceptions of mentoring relationships. *Journal of Vocational Behavior, 51*, 29–42.

Fielden, S. L., Davidson, M. J., & Sutherland, V. J. (2009). Innovations in coaching and mentoring: Implications for nurse development leadership. *Health Services Management Research, 22*, 92–99.

Fox, V. J., Rothrock, J. C., & Skelton, M. (1992). The mentoring relationship. *Association of Perioperative Registered Nurses Journal, 56*(5), 858, 860–862.

Freeman, S. (2004, June 12). *Effective mentoring skills for nurse practitioners.* Presented at the American Academy of Nurse Practitioners Symposium, New Orleans, Louisiana.

Friedman, P. K., Arena, C., Atchison, K., Beemsterboer, P. L., Farsai, P., Giusti, J. B. et al. (2004). Report of the ADEA's President's Commission on Mentoring. *Journal of Dental Education, 68*(3), 390–396.

Galbraith, M. W., & Zelenak, B. S. (1991). Adult learning methods and techniques. In M. W. Galbraith (Ed.), *Facilitating adult learning* (pp. 103–133). Malabar, FL: Krieger.

Gefke, P. (1999). *CHLA mentoring program trainer's guide.* Los Angeles, CA: Gefke International. Cited in Beecroft, P. C., Santner, S., Lacy, M. L., Kunzman, L., & Dorey, F. (2006). New graduate nurses' perceptions of mentoring: Six-year programme evaluation. *Journal of Advanced Nursing, 55*(6), 736–747.

Gibson, D. E. (2004). Role models in career development: New directions for theory and research. *Journal of Vocational Behavior, 65*, 134–156.

Godshalk, V. M., & Sosik, J. J. (2000). Does mentor-protégé agreement on mentor leadership behavior influence the quality of a mentoring relationship? *Group & Organization Management, 25*(3), 291–317.

Godshalk, V. M., & Sosik, J. J. (2003). Aiming for career success: The role of learning goal orientation in mentoring relationships. *Journal of Vocational Behavior, 63*, 417–437.

Golian, L. M., & Galbraith, M. W. (1996). Effective mentoring programs for professional library development. In D. Williams & E. Garten (Eds.), *Advances in library administration and organization* (pp. 95–124). Greenwich, CT: JAI Press.

Greene, M. T., & Puetzer, M. (2002). The value of mentoring: A strategic approach to retention and recruitment. *Journal of Nursing Care Quality, 17,* 63–70.

Greenhaus, J. H., Callanan, G. A., & Godshalk, V. M. (2000). *Career management.* Fort Worth, TX: Dryden Press.

Gregorc, A. F. (1985). *Gregorc style delineator.* Columbia, CT: Gregorc Associates.

Grossman, S. (2005). Developing leadership through shadowing a leader in health care. In H. Feldman & M. Greenberg (Eds.), *Educating nurses for leadership* (pp. 266–278). New York: Springer Publishing.

Grossman, S., & Valiga, T. (2005). *The new leadership challenge: Creating the future of nursing* (2nd ed.). Philadelphia: F.A. Davis.

Hackman, R. J. (1992). Group effectiveness in organizations. In D. M. Dunnette & L. M. Hough (Eds.), *Handbook of industrial and organizational psychology* (Vol. 3, pp. 199–267). Palo Alto, CA: Consulting Academic Press.

Hafford-Letchfield, T., & Chick, N. (2006). Talking across purposes: The benefits of an interagency mentoring scheme for managers working in health and social care settings in the UK. *Work Based Learning in Primary Care, 4,* 13–24.

Halatin, T. J., & Knotts, R. E. (1982). Becoming a mentor: Are the risks worth the rewards? *Supervisory Management, 27*(2), 27–29.

Hargrove, R. (2000). *Masterful coaching fieldbook.* San Francisco: Jossey-Bass.

Hauer, K. E., Teherani, A., Dechet, A., & Aagaard, E. M. (2005). Medical school students' perceptions of mentoring: A focus-group analysis. *Medical Teacher, 27*(8), 732–739.

Hayes, E. (1998). Mentoring and nurse practitioner student self-efficacy. *Western Journal of Nursing Research, 20,* 521–535.

Healy, C. C., & Welchert, A. J. (1990). Mentoring relations: A definition to advance research and practice. *Educational Researcher, 19*(9), 17–21.

Heller, M. P., & Sindelar, N. W. (1991). *Developing an effective teacher mentor program.* Fastback no. 319. Bloomington, IN: Phi Delta Kappa Educational Foundation.

Hunt, D. M., & Michael, C. (1983). Mentorship: A career training and development tool. *Academy of Management Review, 8,* 475–485.

Hurley, A. E., & Fagenson-Eland, E. A. (1996). Challenges in cross-gender mentoring relationships: Psychological intimacy, myths, rumors, innuendoes, and sexual harassment. *Leadership & Organization Development Journal, 17,* 42–49.

Kahn, J. S., & Greenbaltt, R. M. (2009). Mentoring early-career scientists for HIV research careers. *American Journal of Public Health, 99,* S37–S42.

Kalisch, B. J., Falzette, L., & Cooke, J. (2005). Group e-mentoring: A new approach to recruitment into nursing. *Nursing Outlook, 53,* 1899–1205.

Kemp, B. J. (2005). *Ancient Egypt: Anatomy of a civilization.* Boca Raton, FL: Routledge.

Kochan, F. K., & Trimble, S. B. (2000). From mentoring to co-mentoring: Establishing collaborative relationships. *Theory into Practice, 39*(1), 20–28.

Kram, K. E. (1983). Phases of the mentoring relationship. *Academy of Management Journal, 26,* 608–625.

Kram, K. E. (1985). *Mentoring at work: Developmental relationships in organizational life.* Glenview, IL: Scott Foresman.

Kram, K. E., & Hall, D. T. (1996). Mentoring in a context of diversity and turbulence. In E. E. Kossek & S. Lobel (Eds.), *Managing diversity: Human resource strategies for transforming the workplace* (pp. 108–136). Cambridge, MA: Blackwell.

Larkin, G. L. (2003). Mapping, modeling, and mentoring: Charting a course for professionalism in graduate medical education. *Cambridge Quarterly of Healthcare Ethics, 12,* 167–177.

Lester, V., & Johnson, C. (1981). The learning dialogue. In J. Fried (Ed.), *Education for student development* (pp. 49–56). New Directions for Student Services, No. 15. San Francisco: Jossey-Bass.

Levinson, D. J., Darrow, C. M., Klein, E. G., Levinson, M. H., & McKee, B. (1978). *The seasons of a man's life.* New York: Knopf.

Lewellen-Williams, C., Johnson, V. A., Deloney, L. A., Thomas, B. R., Goyol, A., & Henry-Tillman, R. (2006). The POD: A new model for mentoring underrepresented minority faculty. *Academic Medicine, 81,* 275–279.

Manz, C., & Sims, H. P., Jr., (1981). Vicarious learning: The influences of modeling on organizational behavior. *Academy of Management Review, 6,* 105–113.

McCadden, L. (2003). Perfect partnerships: Mentor program lets nursing students and professional learn from one another. *Advance for Nurses, New England, 9,* 23, 38.

MentorNet. (2007). *Success sustained by study: A documentation of MentorNet's growth and a summary of research findings—October 2007.* Retrieved May 24, 2010, from http://www.MentorNet.net/

Miller, L. C., Devaney, S. W., Kelly, G. L., & Kuehn, A. F. (2008). E-mentoring in public health nursing practice. *The Journal of Continuing Education in Nursing, 39*(9), 394–399.

Mills, J., Lennon, D., & Francis, K. (2006). Mentoring matters: Developing rural nurses knowledge and skills. *Collegian, 13*(3), 32–36.

Mullen, E. (1994). Framing the mentoring relationship in an information exchange. *Human Resource Management Review, 4,* 257–281.

Murray, M. (1991). *Beyond the myths and magic of mentoring: How to facilitate an effective mentoring program.* San Francisco: Jossey-Bass.

Myers, I. B., & McCaulley, M. H. (1985). *Manual: A guide to the development and use of the Myers-Briggs type indicator.* Palo Alto, CA: Consulting Psychologists Press.

National Academy of Sciences, National Academy of Engineering, Institute of Medicine. (1997). *Adviser, teacher, role model, friend: On being a mentor to students in science and engineering.* Washington, DC: National Academies Press.

Noe, R. A. (1988). An investigation of the determinants of successful assigned mentoring relationships. *Personnel Psychology, 41,* 457–479.

Nolinske, T. (1995). Multiple mentoring relationships facilitate learning during fieldwork. *American Journal of Occupational Therapy, 49*(1), 39–43.

Norrell, J. E., & Ingoldsby, B. (1991). Surviving academic isolation: Strategies for success. *Family Relations, 40,* 345–347.

Packard, B. W.-L. (2003). Web-based mentoring: Challenging traditional models to increase women's access. *Mentoring & Tutoring, 11*(1), 53–65.

Paterson, M., McColl, M., & Paterson, J. A. (2004). Preparing allied health students for fieldwork in smaller communities. *Australian Journal of Rural Health, 12,* 32–33.

Phillips, L. L. (1977). *Mentors and protégés: A study of the career development of women managers and executives in business and industry.* Unpublished PhD dissertation, University of California Los Angeles.

Pololi, L. H., & Knight, S. (2005). Mentoring faculty in academic medicine: A new paradigm? *Journal of General Internal Medicine, 20*, 866–870.

Pololi, L. H., Knight, S., Dennis, K., & Frankel, R. M. (2002). Helping medical school faculty realize their dreams: An innovative, collaborative mentoring program. *Academic Medicine, 77*(5), 377–384.

Ragins, B. R., & Cotton, J. L. (1993). Gender and willingness to mentor in organizations. *Journal of Management, 19*, 97–111.

Ragins, B. R., & Cotton, J. L. (1999). Mentor functions and outcomes: A comparison of men and women in formal and informal relationships. *Journal of Applied Psychology, 84*, 529–550.

Ragins, B. R., & McFarlin, D. B. (1990). Perceptions of mentor roles in cross-gender mentor relationships. *Journal of Vocational Behavior, 37*, 321–340

Ragins, B. R., & Scandura, T. A. (1994). Gender differences in expected outcomes of mentoring relationships. *Academy of Management Journal, 37*, 957–971.

Ragins, B. R., & Scandura, T. A. (1997). The way we were: Gender and the termination of mentoring relationships. *Journal of Applied Psychology, 82*, 321–339.

Ramsey, D. E., Thompson, J. C., & Braithwaite, H. (1994). Mentoring: A professional commitment. *Journal of the National Black Nurses Association, 7*(1), 68–76.

Rideout, S. (2006). Mentoring: Guided by the light. *PT Magazine, 14*(1), 42–48.

Roberts, A. (1999). The origins of the term mentor. *History of Education Society Bulletin, 64*, 313–329.

Rockman, P., Salach, L., Gotlib, D., Cord, M., & Turner, T. (2004). Shared mental health care: Model for supporting and mentoring family physicians. *Canadian Family Physician, 50*, 397–402.

Scandura, T. A. (1998). Dysfunctional mentoring relationships and outcomes. *Journal of Management, 24*, 449–467.

Shea, G. (1995). Can a supervisor mentor? *Supervision, 56*(11), 3.

Smith, L. S., McAllister, L. E., & Snype Crawford, C. (2001). Mentoring benefits and issues for public health nurses. *Public Health Nursing, 18*(2), 101–107.

Sprecher, S. (1992). Social exchange perceptions on the dissolution of close relationships. In T. L. Orbuch (Ed.), *Close relationship loss* (pp. 47–66). New York: Springer-Verlag.

Standing Committee on Postgraduate Medical and Dental Education. (1998). *An enquiry into mentoring: Supporting doctors and dentists at work*. London: Standing Committee on Postgraduate Medical and Dental Education.

Stewart, S., & Carpenter, C. (2009). Electronic mentoring: An innovative approach to providing clinical support. *International Journal of Therapy and Rehabilitation, 16*(4), 199–206.

Swoboda, M. J., & Millar, S. B. (1986). Networking-mentoring: Career strategy of women in academia administration. *Journal of the National Association for Women Deans, Administrators, and Counselors in Washington, D.C., 50*, 8–13.

Thibaut, J. W., & Kelley, H. H. (1959). *The social psychology of groups*. New York: Wiley.

Thomas, K. W., & Kilmann, R. H. (1991). *Thomas-Kilmann conflict mode instrument*. Tuxedo, NY: Xicom.

Thomas, K. W., & Thomas, G. F. (1991). *Power base inventory*. Tuxedo, NY: Xicom.

Tobin, M. J. (2004). Mentoring: Seven roles and some specifics. *American Journal of Respiratory and Critical Medicine, 170*(2), 114–117.

Verdajo, T. (2002). Mentoring: A model method. *Nursing Management, 33*(8), 15–16.

Wanberg, C. R., Welsh, E. T., & Hezlett, S. A. (2003). Mentoring research: A review and dynamic process model. In G. R. Ferris & J. J. Martocchio (Eds.), *Research in personnel and human resources management* (Vol. 22, pp. 39–124). Oxford, UK: Elsevier.

Wasserstein, A. G., Quistberg, D. A., & Shea, J. A. (2007). Mentoring at the University of Pennsylvania: Results of a faculty survey. *Journal of General Internal Medicine, 22*, 210–214.

Wilson, J. A., & Elman, N. S. (1990). Organizational benefits of mentoring. *Academy of Management Executive, 4*, 88–93.

Woodrow, P. (1994). Mentorship: Perceptions and pitfalls for nursing practice. *Journal of Advanced Nursing, 19*, 812–818.

Wright-Harp, W., & Cole, P. A. (2008). A mentoring model for enhancing success in graduate education. *Contemporary Issues in Communication Science and Disorders, 35*, 4–16.

Zachery, L. J. (2002). The role of the teacher as mentor. *New Directions for Adult and Continuing Education, 93*, 27–38.

Zagumny, M. J. (1993). Mentoring as a tool for change: A social learning perspective. *Organization Development Journal, 11*, 43–48.

Zey, M. G. (1984). *The mentor connection.* Homewood, IL: Dow Jones-Irwin.

Zey, M. G. (1985). Mentor programs: Making the right moves. *Personnel Journal, 64*, 53–57.

ONE

Case Study One

Using Multiple Models of Mentoring

Daniel J. O'Shea and Linda S. Lloyd

INTRODUCTION

Multiple models of mentoring exist, some of which are modifications of classic mentoring models; others have been facilitated by new technologies that allow mentoring to take place across geographic areas. Mentoring models include classic mentoring, peer mentoring, group mentoring, multiple mentor model, preceptorship, shadowing, coaching, role modeling, and distance mentoring.

Additionally, according to Ragins, Cotton and Miller (2000), mentoring can be either informal or formal. The authors describe informal mentoring as a mutually negotiated mentoring relationship in which the mentee selects the mentor because they are viewed as a role model, have similar professional interests, or share common personal characteristics. Informal mentorships are distinguished from formal mentorships in that they are not monitored by an external entity; the content of meetings is not defined and the partnership lasts for the length of time desired by the mentee and mentor. In a formal mentoring relationship, the mentee and mentor have been matched by their organization or an external entity and the parameters of the mentoring relationship have been established to meet organizational needs. In formal mentoring the time frame for the mentoring is also usually established. Formal mentorships often include the exchange of specific information and training, and the relationship generally lasts between 6 months to 1 year.

We describe here the use of multiple models of mentoring that have been used with staff in the public health arena, specifically service planning for Ryan White-funded HIV/AIDS services and a private not-for-profit health care foundation. The authors use the mentoring process for a Health Planner/Analyst position within a County Health Department as an example to highlight their shared mentoring techniques of formal and informal, classic and multiple mentoring, coaching, shadowing, role modeling and peer mentoring.

ORGANIZATIONAL CONTEXT

The health planner/analyst is tasked to perform a variety of planning functions related to care and treatment services for people living with HIV/AIDS (PLWH/A) and in support of the HIV Health Services Planning Council. Duties include gathering and analyzing information to inform the Planning Council process; conducting community outreach, education and group facilitation to encourage increased community and consumer (PLWH/A) involvement in the process; developing service descriptions, performance indicators and outcomes; providing logistical support for meetings of the HIV Planning Council and its committees and task forces, including minute taking and mailings; developing budget spreadsheets for planning purposes; and assisting with grant applications. Required education and/or experience for the job includes a bachelor's degree from an accredited college or university, with major coursework in public health, social services, business/public administration or closely related field and 1 year of professional work experience in the field of health/social service planning or related areas. Additional verifiable qualifying experience may be substituted for the educational requirement on a year-for-year basis. Two years of progressively responsible experience in HIV/AIDS program management, coordination, planning or evaluation are desired.

Organizationally, the health planner/analyst reports to the Ryan White Project Manager (Senior Health Planner), who supervises all Planning Council Support Staff (PCSS). PCSS include four health planners, one administrative assistant and one community liaison. The project manager is responsible for recruiting, hiring, and training all PCSS and provides staff and team leadership. He develops the PCSS Work Plan to ensure appropriate staff and team participation and directs activities of all PCSS, including coordination and oversight of all required planning activities for Ryan White-funded HIV/AIDS care and treatment services, annual needs assessment, priority setting and budget allocations processes. The project manager has over 20 years of experience in planning and providing community services, and 12 years experience as program manager.

After hiring, the first step toward mentorship for the new health planner begins with a general all-day orientation for all new employees to the County and Public Health Services. The second day's agenda includes a brief welcome meeting with the project manager, then a walkthrough with the project manager around the health services facility and the HIV/AIDS and STD branch offices to introduce the health planner to other key staff and provide a brief overview of their various functions, particularly as it may relate to the work of PCSS and planning. The project manager ushers the new employee to their assigned office space, provides information or contacts on how to set up their computer, e-mail and phone, how to navigate in the computer shared drive, a list of who to call when you need help (e.g., the computer help desk) and then allows the new hire a few minutes to settle in.

Next on the agenda is a longer one-on-one meeting with the project manager. This meeting includes a general overview by the project manager of the Ryan White HIV/AIDS Treatment Modernization Act, Planning Council responsibilities versus County responsibilities, and the relationship between the Planning Council and the County. Hard copies of the following are provided: welcome letter from the branch chief, building map, branch organizational chart and phone list, work-related policies and procedures (start and end time, breaks, etc.), 3-year Comprehensive Plan for Services for PLWH/A, which includes a mission statement, vision statement, goals and objectives, and a description of the structure of the Planning Council and committee roles and responsibilities, Planning Council Member Manual, most recent Ryan White Part A grant application, Planning Council Primer, and a list of Internet links (including the federal Health Resources and Services Administration HIV/AIDS Bureau Web site and the Centers Disease Control and Prevention Web site) and Ryan White manuals. The health planner is instructed to add these links to the "Favorites" on her/his computer. Along with the hard-copy resource documents provided, these form the basis of her/his "Mental Desktop." The "Mental Desktop" encompasses resources needed to carry out their job and stay current with any changes.

The health planner is encouraged to spend time within the next week reviewing these materials. A schedule is set up between the project manager and the health planner for weekly one-on-one meetings. The project manager conveys that he has an "open door" policy and, if s/he has any questions, s/he must feel free to stop by. Next, a schedule of the weekly PCSS team meetings, Planning Council, Planning Council committees and other relevant community meetings or activities is distributed. The project manager notes which meetings are required and encourages the health planner to attend other meetings as feasible to broaden her/his perspective on the planning process and various stakeholders involved. He also notes which meetings or activities other PCSS facilitate or to which they are assigned. Finally, a copy of the PCSS Work Plan is provided, highlighting activities assigned to the new health planner.

Ideally, this one-on-one meeting is followed by a special meeting with the whole PCSS team. Otherwise, this would occur as soon as possible within the next few days. The focus of this meeting is to again review the PCSS Work Plan and schedule, and to map out how the new health planner will shadow the project manager and other members of the PCSS team. Before taking on any solo responsibilities, the new health planner will follow the lead of the project manager or other PCSS currently assigned to a specific task.

ONE-ON-ONE MEETINGS: USING THE CLASSICAL AND COACHING MODELS

Classic mentoring has been defined as a long-term relationship between two individuals, often paired by a supervisor. The mentor has the advanced knowledge, skills, and job experience the organization deems key to the future success of the mentee, and expects the mentor to aid in the development of the mentee's organizational skills and professional network. The mentor teaches, coaches, and provides support and encouragement to the mentee. Other authors see the classic mentoring model as more spontaneous and not one in which mentors and mentees are matched by the organization. What these different perspectives have in common, however, is that the mentor plays a role in facilitating the mentee's professional development by sharing knowledge, skills and networks with the mentee through a relationship built on trust (Grossman, 2007).

Although coaching may be a component within the classical model of mentoring, coaching is itself a distinct model. There are many ways to coach, types of coaching and methods for coaching. Coaching consists of directing, instructing and training a person or group of people to achieve an established goal or develop specific skills. Coaching sessions are typically one-on-one either in-person or over the telephone while training may include seminars, workshops, and supervised practice. Coaching is frequently used in job performance, with the goal of working with the employee to solve performance problems and to improve the work of not only the employee, but also the organization.

Both the classical model and the coaching models of mentoring are employed in mentoring the health planner. The health planner continues to meet with the project manager on a weekly basis. This is used as an opportunity to:

- Review progress with the orientation plan (first few weeks)
- Review progress with overall PCSS Work Plan
- Discuss successes and challenges
- Provide feedback on progress to the Health Planner
- Recognize and acknowledge accomplishments
- Brainstorm strategies to overcome any identified challenges
- Identify, assess and discuss the health planner's skills, individual strengths, types of activities that satisfy and motivate and their relation to specific assignments and the way they could be further developed individually and within the team.

The meetings are collectively used as an opportunity to review effectiveness of communication with the project manager and other PCSS and key staff, understanding of work expectations, any resource needs and opportunities for growth and development. The project manager encourages and values input into the strategies and decisions regarding individual and team work. The health planner's personal professional and educational goals are discussed and s/he is encouraged to develop a personal plan to achieve these. Follow-up action items are identified at each meeting to be addressed or for further discussion at the next meeting. This allows for continued assessment of work and opportunities to improve or grow. The project manager strives to make these closed-door meetings a safe, secure place for these discussions.

TEAM STAFF MEETINGS AND FOLLOW-UP: USING THE GROUP, PEER, AND MULTIPLE MENTORING MODELS

Group mentoring offers an alternative to a one-to-one peer mentoring relationship. Group mentoring involves a group of individuals who engage in a mentoring relationship to achieve specific learning goals. This form of mentoring can help an organization extend its mentoring efforts and reach more people in a timely manner, as well as avoid the perception of favoritism when there are limited numbers of mentors and many potential mentees (Zachary, 2009). Three common forms of group mentoring include facilitated group mentoring, peer group mentoring, and team mentoring.

Facilitated group mentoring allows a number of people to participate in a learning group and to benefit simultaneously from the experience and expertise of a mentor or mentors. Each group participant brings their personal experiences into the conversation, which is facilitated by an individual who is external to the group. The facilitator asks questions to ensure a thought provoking and meaningful dialogue, shares their own personal experiences, provides feedback, and serves as a sounding board for the group.

Peer group mentoring brings together peers with similar learning interests or needs. Peer groups are self-directed and self-managed, with the group members developing their learning agenda and managing the learning process. The goal is that each member's learning needs will be met and each member derives maximum benefit from a peer's knowledge, expertise and experience.

Team mentoring facilitates learning by a team. The individuals making up the team articulate their mutual learning goals and work with one or more mentors who guide them through a deliberate and deliberative process to facilitate their learning. The mentoring process allows the team to be supported and to learn from each other's experience and knowledge.

Each of these three forms of team mentoring is utilized by the organization. Each week the project manager convenes a meeting of the whole PCSS team. Similar to the one-on-one meetings, these also focus on the team's progress in achieving the overall PCSS Work Plan. In contrast to the one-on-one meetings, team meetings allow for group interaction, mutual acknowledgement of both individual and team successes, and brainstorming opportunities to address challenges and barriers or improve strategies and outcomes by "bouncing" ideas off each other. The project manager uses this as an opportunity to review the skills and strengths of the team as a composite of the skills and abilities of each individual member. As staff collectively considers their Work Plan and upcoming projects to be accomplished, this information is critical to determining the best match of personnel for each task.

The meeting includes a round-robin which allows each staff person to share what he or she has been working on in the past week, and any issues, including difficulties or frustrations, as well as accomplishments, with opportunity for their peers to offer feedback or share their own best practices for success, sometimes using the group to work collectively toward a solution. If an extensive discussion is expected, the item may be placed on the meeting agenda in advance through consultation with the project manager or by request at the beginning of the meeting. At times, a special meeting may be convened separately to address a specific topic. As with one-on-one meetings, key concepts or action points are captured for further review, discussion or follow-up at the next meeting.

Peer mentoring is also considered to be important in the mentoring process. This form of mentoring relies upon individuals of equal status serving as mentor and mentee, without the hierarchical mentor relationship seen in classic mentoring. However, both models are based upon the mentor and mentee developing a relationship built on trust, through which the mentoring takes place. New health planners are frequently formally paired with seasoned health planners, functioning as peer coaches to assist in their orientation and assigned Work Plan activities. On a routine basis, all health planners are encouraged to act as peer coaches to each other to utilize to advantage the varying knowledge, talents and strengths of the individual team members. The interactive process fosters mutual support through sharing of best practices and problem-solving.

In addition, the new health planner is advised to seek out other team members with more experience for advice and consultation with challenges so they receive mentoring on specific issues from the person most skilled in the issue. This approach reflects the multiple mentor model, which is based on the premise that mentoring can take place simultaneously across several people, with a different type of mentor to assist with meeting the different needs of the mentee.

ENGAGING COMMUNITY STAKEHOLDERS, GROUP FACILITATION, AND PARTICIPATION: SHADOWING AND ROLE MODELING

Shadowing provides the opportunity for an individual to observe a person in a field of interest go about their daily work. The observer will see firsthand the work environment, employability and occupational skills in practice, the value of professional training and potential career options. Shadowing also allows the observer to ask questions while the person is actually working and to investigate their assumptions about that particular field of work.

Many times, but not always, the individual who is to be shadowed by the mentee is also a role model for the mentee. A role model is a person who serves as an example and whose behavior is emulated by others. Role modeling is commonly seen in the health professions, where established and knowledgeable individuals in the field teach by example; that is, they demonstrate the appropriate behaviors and skills for that specific specialty or field. Research has shown that role models are an important factor in shaping the values, attitudes, behavior, and ethics of medical trainees (Wright, Kern, Kolodner, Howard, & Brancati, 1998).

Building trust and providing clear, consistent communication and information are cornerstones to a successful community planning process. Using the schedule of Planning Council, Planning Council committees and other relevant community meetings or activities distributed by the project manager and/or outlined by the PCSS Work Plan and weekly team meetings, the new health planner is instructed to shadow the project manager and/or seasoned health planners and carefully observe and model their interactions and work produced (previous reports) to become adept at performing the following integral community planning functions:

- Gathering, organizing, analyzing, and disseminating data and information to inform HIV planning processes
- Preparing and presenting timely reports and documentation as required or requested, ensuring accuracy, clarity, and a professional user-friendly format
- Establishing effective and cooperative working relationships with members of the public representing diverse health issues, experiences, cultures and backgrounds, contractors, service providers and government officials
- Informing, educating and facilitating community groups and planning committees, including review of data and eliciting recommendations in a clear and nonjudgmental manner
- Providing subject matter expertise and assistance for HIV/AIDS service planning, frequently acting as liaison with community health

service providers, other public, government and private agencies, and community groups

▪ Exercising appropriate judgment in answering questions and releasing information; communicating effectively with a variety of individuals representing diverse cultures and backgrounds and functioning calmly in situations which require a high degree of sensitivity, tact and diplomacy.

Opportunities are created at one-on-one and PCSS Team meetings in which the new health planner can review the observed or documented appropriate behavior, processes or informational format for these activities with the project manager and seasoned health planners, and discuss the background and rationale. New health planners are also afforded the opportunity to role-play activities and presentations at PCSS team meetings in order to gain more confidence for public interactions, participation and presentations, and to receive feedback from their peers in a safer, more comfortable setting. Typically, for community meeting or needs assessment focus groups, the new health planner will function as the recorder, transcribing notes of key points made by participants on a flip chart, while closely observing how the meeting is facilitated by the project manager or seasoned health planner. Eventually, the new health planner will be provided the opportunity to model the behavior by cofacilitating and then taking over full facilitation while the project manager or seasoned health planner then functions as recorder. The latter are able to provide constructive feedback on the new health planner's performance.

In the same way, the new health planner is given written documents and tools previously created to model while updating, modifying or creating new written reports, minutes and tools based upon new analysis or new data. These are reviewed in one-on-one meetings with the project manager and assessed for accuracy, completeness and clarity.

WORKING WITH PLANNING COUNCIL AND COMMITTEE CHAIRS: ADDITIONAL OPPORTUNITIES FOR MULTIPLE MENTORING MODEL

The Planning Council has eight standing committees and may form additional ad hoc committees from time to time to address specific issues and needs. This structure is designed to not only assist the Planning Council in achieving its federally mandated responsibilities under the Ryan White Treatment Modernization Act, but is also the primary vehicle for implementation and oversight of the 3-year Comprehensive Plan. All are supported by a health planner, who also provides subject matter expertise. As a result, much of the work of individual health planners takes place in meetings in the community away from the rest of PCSS. Each of these committees is chaired by a member of the Planning Council, consumers or providers who represent a wide variety of experience, skills and perspectives. The committee chairs typically develop a close working relationship with the assigned health planner, affording other unique opportunities for mentoring relationships depending on the background of the chair (e.g., PLWH/A, mental health provider, primary care provider, HIV researcher, medical case management provider, community clinic provider). As part of the assessment and evaluation of individual health planners, the project manager relies on candid feedback routinely solicited from Planning Council and committee chairs to help assess performance of the health planner in supporting committee work.

FEEDBACK LOOP

The combination of mentoring opportunities and models offered through one-on-one meetings, team staff meetings, follow-up by peers, preparing reports and presentations, engaging community stakeholders, group facilitation and work with Planning Council and committee chairs provides a continuous multi-faceted feedback loop to the health planner. This information enables her/him to build an ever-expanding base of knowledge and skills; continually assess strengths and progress; address often unique challenges and barriers; improve plans, products, services and service systems; and ultimately grow personally and professionally.

PROGRAM SUCCESSES

Over the course of 12 years, over 10 individuals have been mentored using this process. Several have successfully moved on to other higher level responsibilities within the County or other public health programs in the region or across the nation. The local planning and needs assessment processes and community-based responses supported by these staff have been cited as a model in the State of California and across the nation, and allowed the local jurisdiction significant success in competing for federal funds.

The greatest example of the success of this program was a young woman who worked in the program for 6 1/2 years, beginning at half-time in the Ryan White Health Planner position and half-time in an HIV prevention program. Fully using this mentoring model in working with the project manager, she progressively assumed significant leadership and analytical responsibilities in planning public health services for PLWH/A. Within 2 years, she became a Ryan White Planner full-time. Extremely competent, organized, eager and able to learn, absorb and interpret new and complex information, and self-motivated to work independently or as a team player, she easily transitioned within the next year to the relatively new position of lead health planner/analyst, proving to be an invaluable asset to the project manager, county and the community. She in turn used the mentoring model to assist the project manager in development of new staff. Her professional skills and strengths included: responsible, dependable, flexible, self-starter and team player; excellent oral and written communication skills; research and analytical skills with attention to detail and ability to understand and easily absorb complex new data and information; high quality and quantity of work; supervisory and leadership skills; and commitment and dedication to public health in her work with the HIV community. Her outstanding interpersonal communication skills with various community stakeholders, including consumers, community members, providers and County staff engendered universal respect and admiration.

Significant accomplishments included effective leadership and management of the annual community-based planning process to assure quality services for PLWH/A. She coordinated local comprehensive needs assessments every other year, and organized and analyzed quantitative and qualitative data generated through these efforts. She produced or researched and compiled other complex data sets required for planning purposes (epidemiology, service utilization, service outcomes, treatment modalities and protocols, unit cost, etc.), identified key findings and created user-friendly summaries. She used her own initiative to develop well-received tools and exercises on how to interpret data for planning, targeted and tailored to groups of stakeholders with varying degrees of competency.

The community acknowledged her efforts on their behalf with a nomination in 2005 in the area of public policy and planning for the highest award given in the metropolitan area for outstanding achievement "in the struggle against the HIV/AIDS epidemic in our community." She also received the first Certificate of Appreciation from the HIV Consumer Committee for her efforts to educate and encourage involvement by PLWH/A in planning for services.

In her tenure as health planner/lead health planner she gained significant experience, expertise and skills in the public health care services and planning arena. She left the County to pursue a Master's in Public Health degree. After graduation, she went to work as a Prevention Officer on a project to provide HIV/AIDS-related technical assistance services in other countries. She presently works as a regional support manager for a national demonstration program, serving as liaison to community alliances across the nation to improve health care quality and reduce disparities.

REFERENCES

Grossman, S. C. (2007). *Mentoring in nursing*. New York: Springer Publishing Company.

Ragins, B. R., Cotton, J. L., & Miller, J. S. (2000). Marginal mentoring: The effects of type of mentor, quality of relationship, and program design on work and career attitudes. *Academy of Management Journal, 43*(6), 1177–1194.

Wright, S. M., Kern, D. E., Kolodner, K., Howard, D. M., & Brancati, F. L. (1998). Attributes of excellent attending-physician role models. *New England Journal of Medicine, 339*, 1986–1993.

Zachary, Lois J. (2009). *Group mentoring*. Retrieved November 10, 2009, from http://humanresources.about.com/od/coachingmentoring/a/group_mentoring.htm

TWO

Mentoring Faculty for Success

Mentoring faculty in the health professions may be particularly critical to the engagement and retention of junior professionals in academia. As indicated in previous chapters, effective mentoring has been found to be associated with increased earning potential, greater career satisfaction, increased productivity, and an upward career trajectory (Morzinski, Diehr, Bower, & Simpson, 1996; Neumayer, Levinson, & Putnam, 1995; Palepu et al., 1998; Pololi, Knight, Dennis, & Frankel, 2002; Rimm, 1999; Roberts, 1997; Rogers, Holloway, & Miller, 1990; Stange & Hekelman, 1990). These rewards may be particularly important in health professions in which burnout rates and rates of dissatisfaction are high, such as in academic medicine and basic science (Deckard, Hicks, & Hamory, 1992; Lowenstein, Fernandez, & Crane, 2007; Schindler et al., 2006; Shanafelt, Sloan, & Habermann, 2003; Whippen & Canellos, 1991). However, it is in these same fields that the unavailability of appropriate mentors may be greatest. In medicine, for example, senior clinical and basic science faculty may be less willing or less able to take on the responsibilities of mentoring others because of increased administrative and clinical responsibilities (Carroll, 1993; Faxon, 2002), decreased institutional support and rewards for mentoring, and increased pressure to secure the decreasing grant funding available for research (Ludmerer, 1999; Papp & Aron, 2000). A relatively low proportion of doctoral-trained nurses is committed to an academic career (American Association of Colleges of Nursing, 1999); this, together with the retirement of aging nursing faculty, has serious implications for the ability of more junior faculty to identify potential mentors and to attain tenure (Records & Emerson, 2003).

Despite the critical importance of mentoring faculty, and although a significant proportion of faculty in the health professions report having been mentored, relatively few data are available relating to the details of the mentoring process. As an example, between one-third and one-half of surveyed medical school faculty report having been mentored (Palepu et al., 1998; Ramanan, Phillips, Davis, Silen, & Reede, 2002), but published reports often fail to specify whether the mentoring was in the context of formal or informal programs and the duration of these programs. Additionally, reports that are available rarely provide an evaluation of the program over an extended period of time and rarely, if ever, address the impact of such programs on faculty success in all of the varied domains in which faculty are expected to demonstrate achievement—research, teaching, and service.

This chapter first reviews the theoretical underpinnings used in various mentoring programs for which there are published reports, that is, the process that can be used to successfully mentor junior faculty and the context of that mentoring. The chapter then examines the structure of various programs that have been implemented.

THEORETICAL UNDERPINNINGS

The learning theory is relevant to mentoring faculty members' approach to the mentoring of more junior faculty members, to their mentees' development of their own teaching, and to the development and evaluation of a mentoring program itself. (This latter topic is the focus of Chapter 5.) Mentors are expected to have adequate skills to mentor junior faculty; they and their junior faculty mentees are often expected to teach students at levels ranging from the undergraduate to the postgraduate. All too often, however, neither the mentors nor the mentees received adequate preparation for the teaching tasks before them (Clark et al., 2004; Pololi et al., 2001). Indeed, it is often assumed, erroneously unfortunately, that a faculty member who has content expertise necessarily possesses teaching expertise as well and/or that the faculty member's "on-the-job" teaching experiences in the professional academic environment provide sufficient preparation to teach effectively (Wilkerson & Irby, 1998). Although the learning theory may provide the framework for faculty development programs, it appears to be the exceptional program (Pololi et al., 2001), rather than the usual, that focuses on the needs of the teaching faculty and acquaints them with a theoretical framework for their approach to teaching. Many of the published reports relating to faculty mentoring programs fail to specify the theoretical framework that served as the basis for the programs' development (e.g., Tracy, Jagsi, Starr, & Tarbell, 2004; Wingard, Garman, & Reznik, 2004) and, in some cases, it is unclear whether the program was developed with any theory in mind.

Faculty mentoring and/or development programs have relied on one or more of the following theories: adult education theory, critical reflection/transformational learning theory, Rogerian theory, and Erikson's stage theory of development. Each theory is discussed in turn in the context of faculty mentoring. It is important to note that a number of these theories are also relevant to the mentoring of students, which is the focus of the Chapter 3.

Adult Education Theory

Andragogy and self-directed learning have been called the "pillars of adult learning theory" and "two of the foundational theories of adult learning" (Merriam, 2001, p. 3). It is not surprising, then, that they have been used often as the foundation for medical faculty development and mentoring programs (Carroll, 1993; Pololi et al., 2001; Pololi & Knight, 2005; Pololi et al., 2002).

Although *andragogy* was first proposed as a theory of adult learning (Knowles, 1970), it was later viewed more as an approach to or technique of teaching (J. Davenport & J. A. Davenport, 1985; Kaufman, 2003). The concept of andragogy rests on four basic assumptions: (1) a person moves from dependency toward self-direction as he or she matures; (2) the accumulated experience that comes with maturity serves as a resource for learning; (3) as the individual matures, his or her readiness to learn is increasingly oriented toward the individual's social roles; and (4) increasing maturity is accompanied by an increased orientation toward problem-centered, rather than subject-centered, learning (Knowles, 1970). Later research found that not all adults are self-directed learners (Reiter, Eva, Hatala, & Norman, 2002) and that some children may have qualitatively richer experiences than do some adults (Hanson, 1996). Knowles subsequently revised the view of pedagogy as relevant only to children's learning and andragogy as relevant only to adults to suggest that andragogy and pedagogy exist along a spectrum and the approach to be used was more likely to be defined by the learner's familiarity with the topic at hand than by the age of the learner (Knowles, 1984).

These four basic assumptions later gave rise to seven principles of andragogy, which serve as guidelines for teaching adults who are, to some degree, independent and self-directed. These guidelines provide that learners should

- be provided with a comfortable and safe learning environment
- be involved in the mutual planning of the methods to be used and the content of the curriculum
- be involved in an assessment of their own needs
- be encouraged to formulate their learning objectives
- be encouraged to identify resources and how to best use those resources to achieve their goals
- be supported in their attempts to achieve their learning objectives
- be involved in the evaluation of their own learning (Kaufman, 2003)

Knowles' approach views the learner as independent, autonomous, and oriented toward growth and self-improvement. His approach, however, has been criticized for both its failure to consider the impact of culture and society on the individual (Merriam, 2001; Pratt, 1993) and for its embodi-ment of patriarchal values of separation and division (Brookfield, 1995).

The underlying principles of the andragogic approach to learning are relevant both to the process of mentoring faculty and to the mentored faculty in their efforts to teach their students. They suggest that, in both the mentoring process and the teaching process, learners will be more motivated to learn if they are provided with a safe and comfortable envi-ronment that encourages their active participation in the identification of their needs and objectives and the evaluation of their own progress.

Although not specifically noted in published reports, it appears that the Collaborative HIV Prevention in Minority Communities Program at the Center for AIDS Prevention Studies at the University of California, San Francisco, relied to some extent on an andragogic approach to mentoring junior minority faculty to conduct AIDS-related research. The program focused on the development of skills directly relevant to participants' responsibilities, such as grant writing and manuscript prep-aration; provided mentees with the resources they would need to succeed and encouraged them to identify additional ones; and negotiated with mentees' home institutions to provide them with additional resources to increase the likelihood of their success (Zea & Belgrave, 2009).

Self-directed learning theory reflects the varied philosophical lean-ings of the scholars in the fields. Depending on the scholar's orientation, the primary goal of self-directed learning theory is the development of the learner's capacity to be self-directed (Tough, 1971) or the encourage-ment of social and/or political action (Brookfield, 1995; Collins, 1996). Transformational learning (Mezirow, 1981) has been viewed both as a variant of self-directed learning theory (Merriam, 2001) and, as in this chapter, as a distinct theoretical approach (Brookfield, 1995).

Grow (1991) used self-directed learning theory as the basis for the development of his Staged Self-Directed Learning (SSDL) model. Grow pos-ited that (1) the goal of education is to develop lifelong, self-directed learn-ers; (2) teaching varies in response to the listeners, so that good teaching is situational; (3) the extent to which a learner is self-directed or dependent varies with the situation; (4) there is nothing wrong with being a dependent learner; (5) both dependency and self-direction can be taught and be learned; and (6) a theory can be useful even if it is not right. Accordingly, the SSDL model constructs a matrix based on these assumptions. The extent to which a learner is self-directed varies along a spectrum from stage 1, dependent, to stage 4, self-directed. The function of the teacher/mentor should vary at each of these stages to accommodate the needs of the learner. For example, a stage 1 dependent learner is best matched with a teacher who can be authori-tative and serve as a coach. In contrast, a stage 4 self-directed learner would benefit from having a teacher who serves as a consultant and a delegator.

The relevance of Grow's model to the mentoring process is read-ily apparent. Recall from Chapter 1 that mentoring involves a reciprocal process of learning and teaching between the mentor and mentee. As the mentee develops self-efficacy and becomes increasingly independent, the role of the mentor may evolve into one that is increasingly collegial and is increasingly characterized by negotiation.

Critical Reflection/Transformational Learning

Mezirow's focus on critical reflection and transformational learning (1981, 1991) draws heavily on the work of Jurgen Habermas. Habermas posited that there are three learning domains, each of which corresponds to a different aspect of social existence. Work, involving instrumental action, is concerned with how one controls one's environment. This "way of knowing" is premised on empirical knowledge derived from an analysis of events and objects and the confirmation or refutation of hypotheses based on observations. As such, it is governed by technical rules.

> The second learning domain is that of communicative action, which is governed by binding *consensual* norms, which define reciprocal expectations about behavior and which must be understood and recognized by at least two acting objects. Social norms are enforced through sanctions. Their meaning is objectified in ordinary language communication. While the validity of technical rules and strategies depend on that of empirically true or analytically correct propositions, the validity of social norms is grounded only in the intersubjectivity of the mutual understanding of intentions and secured by the general recognition of obligations. (Habermas, 1971, p. 92)

The third learning domain is that of "emancipatory" action, which refers to knowledge derived from self-reflection. An individual's critical self-reflection will yield insights that he or she can use to recognize the reasons for his or her difficulties. Transformational learning constitutes the process of

> becoming critically aware of how and why the structure of psycho-cultural assumptions has come to constrain the way we see ourselves and our relationships, reconstituting this structure to permit a more inclusive and discriminating integration of experience and acting upon these new understandings. (Mezirow, 1981, p. 6)

This process of critical reflection and modification of meaning is prompted when the learner confronts a situation or new information that is not congruent with previously held beliefs. The learner is forced to engage in a reflective thinking process to gain meaning from the information or experience (Boyd & Myers, 1988).

In essence, Mezirow's theory explains

> how adult learners make sense or meaning of their experiences, the nature of the structures that influence the way they construe experience, the dynamics involved in modifying meanings, and the way the structures of meanings

themselves undergo changes when learners find them to be dysfunctional. (Mezirow, 1991, p. xii)

Freire's philosophy of praxis (1970, 1973) can be thought of as a transformational learning theory (cf. Glass, 2001). Freire's conception of education was premised on a praxis consisting of "reflection and action upon the world in order to transform it" (Freire, 1970, p. 36). Freire argued that knowledge to guide action could be achieved through a process of focused questioning and analysis; that knowledge would, in turn, be subject to further questioning and analysis (Freire & Faundez, 1992).

Although educators have relied on Freire's philosophy of praxis and theory of liberation of education in their development of educational programs and curricula, including mentoring programs for faculty in academic medicine (Pololi & Knight, 2005), this "methodological appropriation" has been subject to criticism from a number of scholars (Aronowitz, 1993; Glass, 2001). One writer noted that

> the task of this revolutionary pedagogy is not to foster critical consciousness in order to improve cognitive learning, the student's self-esteem, or even to assist in his aspiration to fulfill his human "potential". . . It is to the liberation of the oppressed as historical subjects within the framework of revolutionary objectives that Freire's pedagogy is directed. (Aronowitz, 1993, pp. 11–12)

Although Freire may not have wished his philosophy of praxis to be appropriated by educational systems, it is nonetheless relevant to general education and, here, for both faculty and student mentoring. The integration of cyclical reflection and action into a mentoring program and a mentoring relationship will encourage both the mentor and the mentee to become more self-aware and to examine more fully their identity, attitudes, beliefs, practices, and relations with the external world (Holmes, 2002), to become "reflective practitioners" (Holmes, 2002, p. 78). This may be particularly important if the school administrators wish to attract a more diverse faculty; such reflection may be the springboard for the development among faculty and administrators alike of a political consciousness (Hoffman-Kipp, Artiles, & López-Torres, 2003). One collaborative mentoring program, for example, creatively integrated Freire's philosophy of praxis into its mentoring approach to help medical school faculty develop a recognition of gender and power issues and skills in negotiation and conflict management (Pololi et al., 2002). Exposure of junior faculty members to the concept of praxis through their mentoring program, whatever form that program may take, may help them to become better teachers and researchers.

For example, team teaching and collaborative planning represent two mechanisms that permit both the integration of the concept of praxis and facilitate the development by junior faculty of improved teaching skills. These activities can occur in conjunction with a more senior faculty member, such as in the traditional dyadic mentoring relationship, or with peers, such as in a more collaborative peer mentoring model. This co-planning or co-teaching process necessarily demands that those involved consider the situation, the group, and the artifacts (content) that constitute the focus of the collaborative reflection. As such, the process of reflection becomes embedded in the everyday activities encountered by the mentees; their thinking, action, and reflection must incorporate varied people, concepts, and standards (Hoffman-Kipp et al., 2003).

The adoption of a philosophy of praxis may also influence the nature and method of research within the health professions. As an example, Holmes (2002, p. 77) has suggested that adoption of this perspective by nurses in academia will help them to ground their research in the "real phenomena of the practice world." He further maintains that through this critical reflection, academic nurses will be able to prevent the wholesale "technicization" of the nursing profession to the exclusion of "the hermeneutic and emancipatory aspects of their practice and thought," such as caring, understanding, and intuition (Holmes, 2002, p. 79).

Rogerian Theory

Carl Rogers advocated the establishment of conditions that would facilitate students' development of "inward freedom" (Rogers, 1962, p. 45). This could be accomplished if the teacher (1) presents the student with a real problem that has meaning and relevance to the student, (2) trusts in the capacity of the student to develop his or her own potentiality, (3) accepts and values the worth of each individual student, (4) is empathic and understands how the process of education and learning appears to the student, and (5) provides the necessary resources, including access to other individuals who may contribute to the student's knowledge. He further asserted that the good teacher

> does not set lesson tasks. He does not assign readings. He does not lecture or expound (unless requested to). He does not evaluate and criticize unless the student wishes his judgment on a product. He does not give examinations. He does not set grades. Perhaps this will make it clear that the teacher is not simply giving lip service to a different approach to learning. *He is actually, operationally, giving his students the opportunity to learn to be responsibly free.* (Rogers, 1962, p. 47) (emphasis added)

The ultimate outcome of the successful student-centered teaching process, according to Rogers, is the transformation of both the student and the teacher (Rogers, 1962, 1967).

Rogers' description of these facilitative conditions and the teacher's approach to his or her student exactly mirrors the kinds of environments and mentor characteristics noted in Chapter 1 as most conducive to a successful mentoring relationship. Like Rogers' "good teacher," the "good mentor" must help his or her mentees learn to be responsibly free in their learning and the pursuit of their goals. The bidirectional effect on the teacher and the learner in Rogers' student-centered teaching process is reminiscent of the mutuality involved in the mentor–mentee relationship. Additionally, the integration of this approach into even a traditional dyadic mentoring arrangement between a senior faculty member and one who is junior could potentially reduce the difficulties that may plague such arrangements, such as issues of power, dependency, and transference.

Rogers' emphasis on the teacher's presentation to the student of relevant problems that require solution lays the groundwork for the use of problem-based learning and the presentation to the mentee of challenging opportunities. Providing mentees with an understanding of the Rogerian approach to learning may also support them in their use of problem-based learning with their students in the health professions.

Pololi and colleagues (2002) described a collaborative mentoring program that utilized a Rogerian framework as a basis for its approach. Participating faculty included MD and PhD holders. Individuals participated in a 3-day session that was followed by a 1-day session each month for a period of 6 months. The program, which focused on skills training, career planning, and scholarly writing, used a variety of teaching strategies, including videotaping, role-playing, narrative writing, and reflection.

Erikson's Stages of Development

Erikson theorized that individuals develop and progress through distinct stages of growth over the life course, each characterized by specific tasks that must be learned to acquire the skills necessary to navigate successfully through life's many and varied demands and to progress to the next stage of development. These stages include four preadolescent stages, adolescence (teenage years), early adulthood (20s and 30s), middle age (40s and 50s), and later life (age 60 years and older) (Erikson, 1964, 1968, 1997). Although the stages of development are presumed to be universal, individuals may differ in how they navigate these phases due to variations in personality, culture, life events, and general circumstances.

The stages most relevant to participation in a mentoring relationship, whether as a mentor or as a mentee, are stages 6 through 9. These stages mark the period that begins with young adulthood and extends through the age of 80 or 90 years, when individuals may have retired from their careers but continue to serve as mentors to younger professionals. During *Stage 6, young adulthood*, individuals must develop the capacity to become intimate with and care about others; the antithesis to this intimacy is isolation. Individuals who successfully resolve this conflict acquire the ability to love and exhibit healthy patterns of cooperation and competition in their relations with others. These patterns are critical if one is to function successfully as a professional in the health fields.

Stage 7, *adulthood*, reflects the crisis of generativity versus self-absorption and stagnation. Generativity encompasses procreativity, productivity, and creativity, ushering in new beings (children) as well as new ideas and products. In contrast, those who stagnate remain focused on their own wants and desires, resulting in what Erikson has called "generative frustration" (Erikson, 1997, p. 68). During *Stage 8, old age*, the individual will look back on his or her life with a sense that it has been meaningful and satisfying or a sense of despair at all that has been lost (Erikson, 1951, 1997). The final *Stage 9, gerotranscendence*, corresponds to the 80s and 90s in life and may reflect a conflict between a sense of deepening despair associated with the hurdles, burdens, and losses of older age and basic trust and hope, which gives rise to a continued reason for living (Erikson, 1997).

Other scholars have expanded on Erikson's concepts. As an example, John Kotre (1984, p. 10) defined generativity as "a desire to invest one's substance in forms of life and work that will outlive the self." He hypothesized that there exist four major types of generativity. They include (1) the biological type, which focuses on the bearing and nursing of offspring; (2) the parental type, which emphasizes the nurturing and disciplining of offspring and their initiation into family traditions; (3) the technical type, involving the transmission of knowledge and skills to successors; and (4) the cultural type, which deals with the creation, renovation, and conservation of a symbol system and its transmittal to successors.

Ideally, the establishment of a mentoring program, as well as the selection process for mentors and mentees, should consider the numbers of potential faculty participants at each stage of development. As an example, one would expect a higher prevalence of junior faculty at the stage of young adulthood. Mid-level faculty are more likely to be at a stage of adulthood, whereas senior faculty are more likely to be at the stage of adulthood, old age, or gerotranscendence. However, because individuals vary in how they navigate these phases, this correlation between career level and developmental stage is neither predetermined nor universal. Accordingly, the development of a mentoring program must consider both the extent to which there are available faculty who are in a stage of gerotranscendence and whether the gerotranscendence is of a type that is consistent with the professional responsibilities associated with mentoring, that is, either the technical type or the cultural type.

The Collaborative Mentoring Program of the University of Massachusetts Medical School (Pololi & Knight, 2005; Pololi et al., 2002) appears to be one of the few published mentoring programs that has relied on Erikson's stage model in its development. In formulating this program, program leadership recognized that senior-level faculty at the stage of generativity

> may have a tendency to discount collaborative group peer mentoring models for junior faculty as these do not reflect their own altruistic motivations to mentor. Ideally, we need a structure that honors the altruism of senior faculty and utilizes the benefits and opportunities that this experienced group can offer. (Pololi & Knight, 2005, p. 868)

The program leadership also recognized the contributions that could be made by more junior-level faculty at the stage of young adulthood or early adulthood to not only their own career development but also to the creation of "an environment of support and guidance for achieving career satisfaction and advancement" (Pololi et al., 2002, p. 380) and the facilitation of their membership as "part of a collaborative and collegial team," key goals of the mentoring program. The young adulthood impetus to learn to compromise and sacrifice, to both compete and collaborate, could serve as a springboard for the development of facilitated peer group mentoring. The absence of a formal hierarchical dynamic, such as that reflected in the typical dyadic mentoring model, facilitated the development of intragroup collaboration and collegiality and reduced participants' sense of isolation in the academic environment.

SUMMARY OF THEORETICAL APPROACHES

These varied approaches to understanding adult development and learning share a number of features. First, each postulates a growth trajectory, whether in ongoing learning, the development of relationships, or the development of increasing maturity. Second, each of these approaches identifies the individual adult as the locus of control in decision making, rather than an external force. This is true whether it is in the context of the learning process (Grow), critical reflection (Habermas, Mezirow, & Freire), or navigation through life's many challenges and opportunities (Erikson). Each of these approaches offers insights into the mentoring process and can be used singly or in combination as the foundation of faculty mentoring programs. Table 2.1 provides a summary of these approaches and their potential contribution to the faculty mentoring process.

Just as these approaches share commonalities, so too do they share limitations. Each approach places considerable emphasis on the cognitive aspects of adult learning and fails to address the interaction of emotion and cognition in learning adequately. The relevance of these approaches cross-culturally and the implications of sex and gender identity or role differences are also largely overlooked by each approach.

TABLE 2.1

Summary of Selected Learning Theories and Their Relevance to Mentoring

Theory	Relevance to Mentoring Faculty	Relevance to Mentored Faculty	Examples of Program
Andragogy	Argues for creation of comfortable and safe learning environment Indicates need to include mentee in the process of assessment of needs; development of training plan, career objectives, and career plan; evaluation of progress Supports mentor provision of psychosocial support to mentee	Can be used as an approach to teach their students	Collaborative Mentoring Program, Brody School of Medicine, East Carolina University (Pololi et al., 2001, 2002)
Self-directed learning theory	Places primary responsibility for learning on mentee Encourages mentor to foster increasing skill acquisition and autonomy by mentee	Encourages mentored faculty member to continuously learn to improve skills Provides a foundation for faculty members to encourage students to assume responsibility for their own learning	Collaborative Mentoring Program, Brody School of Medicine, East Carolina University (Pololi et al., 2002)
Critical reflection/ transformational learning theory	Encourages mentor to provide mentee with challenging opportunities Encourages recognition of gender and power issues	Encourages recognition of gender and power issues Supports mentee development of communication and negotiation skills	Collaborative Mentoring Program, Brody School of Medicine, East Carolina University (Pololi et al., 2002)

(Continued)

TABLE 2.1 (Continued)

Summary of Selected Learning Theories and Their Relevance to Mentoring

Theory	Relevance to Mentoring Faculty	Relevance to Mentored Faculty	Examples of Program
Rogerian theory	Encourages mentor to present mentee relevant problems/challenges Supports mentor provision to the mentee of psychosocial support Underscores the need to provide necessary resources and opportunities for the mentee to succeed and assist mentee to develop a professional network	Provides mentee with opportunities for increased self-knowledge and creativity through attempts to resolve problems and address challenges Encourages mentee to use problem-based learning in teaching	Collaborative Mentoring Program, Brody School of Medicine, East Carolina University (Pololi et al., 2001, 2002)
Erikson's stage theory of development	Selection of faculty mentor	Selection of faculty mentee	Collaborative Mentoring Program of the University of Massachusetts Medical School (Pololi & Knight, 2005; Pololi et al., 2002)

MENTORS MENTORING FACULTY TO TEACH

Many, if not most, faculty members in the health professions may be required to have basic teaching skills (Wilkerson & Irby, 1998). Despite this expectation, the mentoring of health professionals often places greater emphasis on mentoring for research. A minority of medical schools offer faculty mentoring or development programs in teaching skills (Clark et al., 2004), and faculty are quickly socialized into a value system that rewards and recognizes research and associated scholarship more highly than teaching (Papp & Aron, 2000; Ramani, 2006).

Nevertheless, efforts to assist mentees in the improvement of their teaching skills can be a focus of the mentoring relationship and/or a component of a larger faculty development program. The School of Medicine of the Medical College of Georgia, for example, specifically notes on its Web site for The Academy of Medical Educators (http://www.mcg.edu/som/ames/faq.html) that mentors help junior faculty to develop their education and teaching skills. The British Medical Council (2003) noted in its publication entitled *Tomorrow's Doctors* that medical practitioners are obligated to teach others, particularly physicians in training; that teaching skills can be learned; and that the teacher serves as a role model for the conduct and standards of his or her trainees. Mentoring in teaching can take several forms including mentor observation of the mentee in actual teaching situations and the provision of feedback to the mentee from these observations; mentor review with the mentee of student evaluations of the teaching; and/or mentee co-teaching with a more experienced and knowledgeable teaching mentor.

Accordingly, it is critical that mentors involved in mentoring faculty to teach understand how individuals actually learn to teach. Research has identified five distinct orientations to learning how to teach (Oosterheert & Vermunt, 2001). These are variously termed survival, closed reproduction, open reproduction, closed meaning, and open meaning.

Individuals oriented to a survival approach to learning how to teach do not appear to experience internal motivation to improve their teaching performance. Problems are defined externally and are often attributed to the student. External information regarding their performance is welcomed when it helps to resolve an already-existing problem.

Individuals who are reproduction oriented, whether open or closed, are focused on the improvement of their performance through the integration of practical information that responds to the questions "How" and "What." Those who have a closed reproduction orientation are not concerned with the meaning behind actions and events but with the acquisition of external information that will help them to resolve an already-existing problem as immediately as possible. They are, however, self-regulative in the improvement of their teaching performance. In contrast, those with an open reproduction orientation rely on external regulation for the improvement of their teaching performance.

In contrast to those who are reproduction oriented, meaning-oriented individuals seek to improve their teaching by expanding their understanding of the teaching and learning processes, including the underlying concepts. Those with a closed-meaning orientation view difficulties as problems of performance and rely on external regulation as the basis of their frame of reference on teaching and learning. In contrast, those with an open-meaning orientation are self-regulative, and problems are viewed as problems of performance and of understanding (Oosterheert & Vermunt, 2001).

Perhaps the most significant difference between those who are survival and reproduction oriented on the one hand and those who are meaning oriented on the other lies in the individuals' willingness to assume risk. Those who are meaning oriented are, in general, more willing to acknowledge and address the possibility that an expansion of their knowledge and understanding may provoke a process of self-evaluation, the reconceptualization of their beliefs, and significant modification of their frame of reference and, as a consequence, bring about fundamental changes in their approach to daily living (Oosterheert & Vermunt, 2001). This process is reminiscent of the goals of transformational learning theory, whereby individuals are transformed through critical reflection and modification of meaning.

MENTORING FACULTY IN RESEARCH

Mentoring faculty in conducting research may pose unique challenges. First, unlike students and postdoctoral fellows, individuals holding faculty appointments may feel that they are not entitled to and cannot ask for support or assistance because of their faculty position (Johnston & McCormack, 1997). Even when they are open to mentoring opportunities and these opportunities are made available, they may experience difficulty assuming the role of mentee while simultaneously serving as faculty (Zea & Belgrave, 2009). Increased competition, demands for greater productivity, and the resulting erosion of collegiality may reduce the ability of new faculty members to meet colleagues (Olsen, 1993).

Reliance on an andragogic approach to overcome these difficulties suggests that the content provided through the mentoring process must be directly relevant to the needs of the mentees. Research has identified the content and skills that are critical to academic career success and that should, accordingly, constitute the focus of mentoring. Many of these content areas are relevant to the development of an academic career that is focused in whole or part on research: conducting research, grant writing, negotiating, organization and committee participation, professional networking, and publishing (Lewellen-Williams et al., 2006).

One example of a faculty mentoring program with a focus on research is that of Pennsylvania State University College of Medicine (Thorndyke, Gusic, & Milner, 2008). This program involved 97 faculty as mentees over a period of 4 years. The 9-month program was designed to assist junior faculty members with their career development, research, clinical practice, and education. Each participating faculty mentee was required to initiate and develop a project that was relevant to his or her career goals; the mentor was to provide guidance on the conduct of the project. Slightly more than one-half (55%) of the faculty mentees focused their project on research, with the remaining mentees developing projects related to education or clinical practice. Mentees' self-assessments suggested that the program was beneficial both in helping them to develop skills in preparing grant proposals and in meeting their career goals. The published report did not provide details of these mentoring relationships.

The peer Collaborative Mentoring Program of the National Center of Leadership in Academic Medicine at East Carolina University is an example of a mentoring program that provides mentees with support in the publication of their research (Pololi, Knight, & Dunn, 2004). Publication is often critical to promotion, the award of tenure, and the award of additional research funds (Hekelman, Gilchrist, Zyzanski, Glover, & Olness, 1995; Jones & Gold, 1998). Participants in the mentoring program included both physicians and nonphysicians with doctoral degrees in other disciplines. The program, which consisted of one 3-day session and six monthly day-long sessions, sought to identify and minimize barriers to writing, increase participants' writing knowledge and skills, develop individual writing strategies, promote positive attitudes toward writing, and facilitate the writing process through peer collaboration and feedback. Each day-long session included facilitation by an experienced writer or editor, feedback from mentors, and 20 minutes of time for free and continuous writing. Each participant was required to develop a formal contract on a monthly basis for the completion of specified goals during the upcoming month. Participant evaluations suggested that the mentoring program resulted in an increase in writing-related confidence and a decrease in writing-related anxiety among the participants.

However, these task-related aspects of mentoring may often be unrelated to mentees' level of satisfaction with the mentoring relationship. A questionnaire study of 3,636 instructors and assistant professors at Harvard Medical School and its 17 affiliated independent hospitals and institutions found that seven specific qualities of the mentor were significantly associated with higher overall satisfaction with mentoring, even after adjusting for sex, ethnicity, and academic rank (Ramanan et al., 2002). These included maintaining contacts, not abusing power, providing advice on professional decisions, helping to establish professional networks, giving guidance on career plans and research, offering advice on research, and providing opportunities to enhance communication skills.

Case Study 2 by Horwitz and colleagues, which follows this chapter, provides an example of a systematic approach to faculty career development through the use of a multiple mentor model that combines both a "cis" and a "trans" approach. The requirement that the mentee develop a Career Development Plan is reflective of an andragogic approach in that it is the mentee who drives the assessment of his or her needs and the development of a training plan, career objectives, and a career plan; of self-directed learning theory in that the primary responsibility for learning is placed directly on the trainee; and of Rogerian theory in that the mentor is charged with the responsibility to provide the resources and opportunities necessary to facilitate the mentee's success.

REFERENCES

American Association of Colleges of Nursing. (1999). *AACN issue bulletin: Faculty shortages intensify nation's nursing deficit.* Retrieved October 29, 2010 from http://www.aacn.nche.edu/publication/issues/IB499WB.htm

Aronowitz, S. (1993). Paulo Freire's radical democratic humanism. In P. McLaren & P. Leonard (Eds.), *Paulo Freire: A critical encounter* (pp. 8–24). London: Routledge.

Boyd, R. D., & Myers, J. G. (1988). Transformative education. *International Journal of Lifelong Education, 7,* 261–284.

British Medical Council. (2003). *Tomorrow's doctors.* Retrieved May 24, 2010, from http://www.gmc-uk.org/education/undergraduate/tomorrows_doctors_2003.asp

Brookfield, S. (1995). Adult learning: An overview. In A. Tuinjman (Ed.), *International encyclopedia of education.* Oxford, UK: Pergamon Press.

Carroll, R. G. (1993). Implications of adult education theories for medical school faculty development programmes. *Medical Teacher, 15*(2/3), 163–170.

Clark, J. M., Houston, T. K., Kolodner, K., Branch, W. T., Jr., Levine, R. B., & Kern, D. E. (2004). Teaching the teachers: National survey of faculty development in departments of medicine in U.S. teaching hospitals. *Journal of General Internal Medicine, 19,* 205–214.

Collins, M. (1996). On contemporary practice and research: Self-directed learning to critical theory. In R. Edwards, A. Hanson, & P. Raggatt (Eds.), *Boundaries of adult learning: Adult learners, education and training* (pp. 109–127). New York: Routledge.

Davenport, J., & Davenport, J. A. (1985). A chronology and analysis of the andragogy debate. *Adult Education Quarterly, 35*(3), 152–159.

Deckard, G. J., Hicks, L. I., & Hamory, B. H. (1992). The occurrence and distribution of burnout among infectious disease physicians. *Journal of Infectious Disease, 165,* 224–228.

Erikson, E. H. (1951). *Childhood and society.* New York: W.W. Norton & Company.

Erikson, E. H. (Ed.). (1964). *Insight and responsibility.* New York: W.W. Norton & Company.

Erikson, E. H. (Ed.). (1968). *Youth and crisis.* New York: W.W. Norton & Company.

Erikson, E. H. (1997). *The life cycle completed.* New York: W.W. Norton & Company.

Faxon, D. P. (2002). The chain of scientific discovery: The critical role of the physician-scientist. *Circulation, 105,* 1857–1860.

Freire, P. (1970). *Pedagogy of the oppressed.* New York: Seabury.

Freire, P. (1973). *Education for critical consciousness.* New York: Seabury.

Freire, P., & Faundez, A. (1992). *Learning to question.* New York: Continuum.

Glass, R. D. (2001). On Paulo Freire's philosophy of praxis and the foundations of liberation education. *Educational Researcher, 30,* 15–25.

Grow, G. O. (1991). Teaching learners to be self-directed. *Adult Education Quarterly, 41,* 125–149.

Habermas, J. (1971). *Knowledge and human interests.* Boston, MA: Beacon Press.

Hanson, A. (1996). The search for a separate theory of adult learning: Does anyone really need andragogy? In R. Edwards, A. Hanson, & P. Raggatt (Eds.), *Boundaries of adult learning: Adult learners, education and training* (pp. 99–108). New York: Routledge.

Hekelman, F. P., Gilchrist, V., Zyzanski, S. J., Glover, P., & Olness, K. (1995). An educational intervention to increase faculty publication productivity. *Family Medicine, 27*(4), 255–259.

Hoffman-Kipp, P., Artiles, A. J., & López-Torres, L. (2003). Beyond reflection: Teacher learning as praxis. *Theory Into Practice, 42*(3), 248–254.

Holmes, C. A. (2002). Academics and practitioners: Nurses as intellectuals. *Nursing Inquiry, 9,* 73–83.

Johnston, S., & McCormack, C. (1997). Developing research potential through a structured mentoring program. Issues arising. *Higher Education, 33,* 251–264.

Jones, R. F., & Gold, J. S. (1998). Faculty appointment and tenure policies in medical sciences: A 1997 status report. *Academic Medicine, 73*(2), 212–219.

Kaufman, D. M. (2003). ABC of learning and teaching in medicine: Applying educational theory in practice. *British Medical Journal, 326,* 213–216.

Knowles, M. S. (1970). *The modern practice of adult education: Andragogy versus pedagogy.* New York: Association Press.

Knowles, M. S. (1984). *The adult learner: A neglected species* (3rd ed.). Houston, TX: Gulf.

Kotre, J. (1984). *Outliving the self: Generativity and the interpretation of lives.* Baltimore, MD: Johns Hopkins University Press.

Lewellen-Williams, C., Johnson, V. A., Deloney, L. A., Thomas, B. R., Goyol, A., & Henry-Tillman, R. (2006). The POD: A new model for mentoring underrepresented minority faculty. *Academic Medicine, 81*(3), 275–279.

Lowenstein, S. R., Fernandez, G., & Crane, L. A. (2007). Medical school faculty discontent: Prevalence and predictors of intent to leave academic careers. *BMC Medical Education, 7,* 37. Retrieved October 29, 2010 from http://www.biomedcentral.com/1472-6920/7/37

Ludmerer, K. M. (1999). *Time to heal: American medical education from the turn of the century to the era of managed care.* Oxford, UK: Oxford University Press.

Merriam, S. B. (2001). Andragogy and self-directed learning: Pillars of adult learning theory. In S. B. Merriam (Ed.), *The new update on adult learning theory* (pp. 3–13). San Francisco, CA: Jossey-Bass.

Mezirow, J. (1981). A critical theory of adult learning and education. *Adult Education Quarterly, 32,* 3–24.

Mezirow, J. (1991). *Transformative dimensions of adult learning.* San Francisco, CA: Jossey-Bass.

Morzinski, J. A., Diehr, S., Bower, D. J., & Simpson, D. E. (1996). A descriptive, cross-sectional study of formal mentoring for faculty. *Family Medicine, 28,* 434–438.

Neumayer, L., Levinson, W., & Putnam, C. (1995). Residents' concerns: Mentors for women in surgery and their effect on career advancement. *Current Surgery, 52,* 163–166.

Olsen, D. (1993). Work satisfaction and stressing the first and third year of academic appointment. *Higher Education, 23*(3), 273–295.

Oosterheert, I. E., & Vermunt, J. D. (2001). Individual differences in learning to teach: Relating cognition, regulation and affect. *Learning and Instruction, 11,* 133–156.

Palepu, A., Friedman, R. H., Barnett, R. C., Carr, P., Ash, A. S., Szalacha, L., et al. (1998). Junior faculty members' mentoring relationships and their professional development in US medical schools. *Academic Medicine, 73,* 318–323.

Papp, K. K., & Aron, D. C. (2000). Reflections on academic duties of medical school faculty. *Medical Teacher, 22*(4), 406–411.

Pololi, L., Clay, M. C., Lipkin, M., Jr., Hewson, M., Kaplan, C., & Frankel, R. M. (2001). Reflections on integrating theories of adult education into a medical school faculty development course. *Medical Teacher, 23*(3), 276–283.

Pololi, L., & Knight, S. M. (2005). Mentoring faculty in academic medicine: A new paradigm? *Journal of General Internal Medicine, 20,* 866–870.

Pololi, L. H., Knight, S. M., Dennis, K., & Frankel, R. M. A. (2002). Helping medical school faculty realize their dreams: An innovative, collaborative mentoring program. *Academic Medicine, 17*(5), 377–384.

Pololi, L., Knight, S., & Dunn, K. (2004). Facilitating scholarly writing in academic medicine: Lessons learned from a collaborative peer mentoring program. *Journal of General Internal Medicine, 19,* 64–68.

Pratt, D. D. (1993). Andragogy after twenty-five years. In S. B. Merriam (Ed.), *Update on adult learning theory: New directions for adult and continuing education* (pp. 15–25). San Francisco, CA: Jossey-Bass.

Ramanan, R., Phillips, R., Davis, R. B., Silen, W., & Reede, J. (2002). Mentoring in medicine: Keys to satisfaction. *American Journal of Medicine, 112,* 336–341.

Ramani, S. (2006). Twelve tips to promote excellence in medical teaching. *Medical Teacher, 28,* 19–23.

Records, K., & Emerson, R. J. (2003). Mentoring for research skill development. *Journal of Nursing Education, 42*(12), 553–557.

Reiter, H. I., Eva, K. W., Hatala, R. M., & Norman, G. R. (2002). Self and peer assessment in tutorials: Application of a relative-ranking model. *Academic Medicine, 77,* 1134–1139.

Rimm, S. (1999). *See Jane win: The Rimm report on how 1,000 girls became successful women.* New York: Crown Publishers.

Roberts, K. (1997). Nurse academics' scholarly productivity: Framed by the system, facilitated by mentoring. *Australian Journal of Advanced Nursing, 14*(3), 5–14.

Rogers, C. R. (1962). Learning to be free (Part two). *Pastoral Psychology, 13*(9), 43–51.

Rogers, C. R. (1967). The facilitation of significant learning. In L. Siegel (Ed.), *Instructions: Some contemporary viewpoints* (pp. 37–54). San Francisco, CA: Chandler.

Rogers, J. C., Holloway, R. L., & Miller, S. M. (1990). Academic mentoring and family medicine's research productivity. *Family Medicine, 22*, 186–190.

Schindler, B. A., Novack, D. H., Cohen, D. G., Yager, J., Wang, D., Shaheen, N. J. et al. (2006). The impact of the changing health care environment on the health and well-being of faculty at four medical schools. *Academic Medicine, 81*(1), 27–34.

Shanafelt, T. D., Sloan, J. A., & Habermann, T. M. (2003). The well-being of physicians. *American Journal of Medicine, 114*, 513–519.

Stange, K. C., & Hekelman, F. P. (1990). Mentoring needs and family medicine faculty. *Family Medicine, 22*, 183–185.

Thorndyke, L. E., Gusic, M., & Milner, R. J. A. (2008). Functional mentoring: A practical approach with multilevel outcomes. *Journal of Continuing Education in the Health Professions, 28*(3), 157–164.

Tough, A. (1971). *The adult's learning projects: A fresh approach to theory and practice in adult learning*. Toronto, Canada: Ontario Institute for Studies in Education.

Tracy, E. E., Jagsi, R., Starr, R., & Tarbell, N. J. (2004). Outcomes of a pilot faculty mentoring program. *American Journal of Obstetrics and Gynecology, 191*, 1846–1850.

Whippen, D. A., & Canellos, G. P. (1991). Burnout syndrome on the practice of oncology: Results of a random survey of 1000 oncologists. *Journal of Clinical Oncology, 9*, 1916–1920.

Wilkerson, L., & Irby, D. M. (1998). Strategies for improving teaching practices: A comprehensive approach to faculty development. *Academic Medicine, 73*(4), 387–396.

Wingard, D. L., Garman, K. A., & Reznik, V. (2004). Facilitating faculty success: Outcomes and cost benefit of the UCSD National Center of Leadership in Academic Medicine. *Academic Medicine, 79*(10), S9–S11.

Zea, M. C., & Belgrave, F. Z. (2009). Mentoring and research capacity-building experiences: Acculturating to research from the perspective of the trainee. *American Journal of Public Health, 99*, S16–S19.

TWO

Case Study Two

The Career Development Plan: A Tool to Improve the Mentored Career Development Experience

Sarah McCue Horwitz, James C. Spilsbury, Klara K. Papp, and Richard Rudick

BACKGROUND

Concerned by the shrinking number of physician scientists and the dearth of clinical research, including patient-oriented research, the Director of the National Institutes of Health (NIH), Harold Varmus, MD, constituted the Director's Panel on Clinical Research in July, 1995 (Goldstein & Brown, 1997; Nathan, 1998). The Panel recommended continuing mentored opportunities in clinical research for medical students, the promotion of clinical research training, the provision of partial salary support for mentors, the inclusion of more physicians on NIH review committees, collaborations across disciplines, and a joint policy between the academic health centers and NIH for the support of clinical research and training (Nathan, 1998).

Progress on these recommendations was subsequently evaluated, with the conclusion that clinical research was adequately supported but that translational research—research at the interface between basic science and clinical application—continued to be underfunded (Nathan & Wilson, 2003). After the appointment of Elias A. Zerhouni, MD, as Director of the NIH in 2002, a series of meetings involving over 300 biomedical experts, produced a plan—the NIH Roadmap for Medical Research—to address the major challenges in biomedical research. Three foci emerged: "new pathways to scientific discovery," "scientific teams of the future," and "re-engineering the clinical research enterprise" (James, 2003; McLellan, 2003; Wang, 2003). The theme of translational research was heavily featured in the NIH Roadmap Initiative and was particularly evident in a new training program designed to produce an interdisciplinary work force (Zerhouni, 2003).

These institutional training programs entitled "Multidisciplinary Clinical Research Career Development Programs" (MCRCDP) (http://grants1.nih.gov/grants/guide/rfa-files/rfa-rm-04-006.html) were designed to support early career scholars from a variety of disciplines engaged in the entire spectrum of clinical research including patient-oriented, translational, clinical investigations, epidemiologic, and natural history research. The program provided 2 to 5 years of support, mandated training in clinical research skills, required multiple mentors, career and educational plans and monitoring/evaluation of program effectiveness, and scholar progress.

The MCRCDPs recognized the importance of mentoring for successful career development, a theme consistent in the academic literature. Since the pioneering work of Levinson and colleagues in the 1970s (Levinson, Darrow, Klein, Levinson, & McKee, 1978), mentors have been conceptualized as "trusted counselors or guides" who help shape the development of the mentee (Hegstad & Wentling, 2004), much as Mentor did for Telemachus (*Webster's Ninth New Collegiate Dictionary*, 1983, p. 742). Mentoring has been characterized by the nature of the relationship (formal vs. informal), the function of the relationship (career development and/or psychosocial), levels of trust, and instrumental activities such as information and skill development. Tools to assess mentoring potential, needs identification grids, lists of mentoring functions and desirable characteristics are available in the literature (Berk, Berg, Mortimer, Walton-Moss, & Yeo, 2005; Cupples, 1999; Erdem & Aytemur, 2008; Rogers, Monteiro, & Nora, 2008; Sands, Parson, & Duane, 1991). Studies with academic faculty suggest that having a satisfying mentoring relationship is related to job satisfaction, lower expectations for leaving the institution, self-efficacy ratings on multiple academic skills, and greater research productivity (Boyle & Boice, 1998; Garman, Wingard, & Reznik, 2001; Wasserstein, Quistberg, & Shea, 2007).

However, as pointed out by Sambunjak, Straus, and Marusić (2006), the evidence base for the importance of mentoring is not strong. This may, in part, be attributable to the reality that while much has been written about the aspects of mentoring that are perceived to be important, there are little data on which aspects of the mentoring process are most beneficial or on techniques/tools/approaches that promote successful mentoring (Levinson et al., 1978). Also, much less attention has been focused on the mentees' responsibilities in the mentoring process (Ludwig & Stein, 2008). Given that, the MCRCDPs required at least two mentors with somewhat different responsibilities (one focused principally on research, with the other focused on the mentee's overall career development), coordinating and overseeing the mentoring relationships posed additional challenges beyond those found in traditional faculty mentoring programs.

CASE-CLEVELAND CLINIC MULTIDISCIPLINARY CLINICAL RESEARCH TRAINING PROGRAM (MCRTP)

Program Structure

The Case-Cleveland Clinic Multidisciplinary Clinical Research Training Program was one of the original seven institutional "K" training programs funded under the previously described announcement. As per the instructions in the Request for Applications, the MCRTP featured: (1) a structured curriculum integrated with the existing courses developed under a Clinical Research Curriculum Award (K30); (2) high quality multidisciplinary translational research; (3) a strong focus on mentoring; (4) a commitment that each K12 scholar would construct a career development plan; and (5) monitoring/evaluating both the mentoring and scholars' career development. The challenges to implementing these features within the MCRTP, however, were considerable. The Case-Cleveland Clinic program was aggressively committed to recruiting educationally (PhD, MD, DDS, DO, DSN, PsyD) and disciplinarily (medicine, arts and sciences, engineering, nursing, dentistry, law) diverse cohorts of scholars. The training program was multi-institutional, involving the major biomedical institutions in Cleveland, Ohio: Case Western Reserve University, the Cleveland Clinic, University Hospitals, MetroHealth System, and the Cleveland Veterans Administration Medical Center. Further, although individual investigators collaborated across these institutions, this was the first training program involving all five institutions. A multidisciplinary advisory committee (MAC) was established, with accomplished clinical investigators from all five institutions, representing the disciplines of medicine, nursing, surgery, mental health, bioethics, social sciences, engineering, dentistry, biostatistics, and epidemiology. The MAC was charged with overseeing the program, including the selection of a multidisciplinary group of scholars.

A multi-institutional Mentoring Committee was formed as a subcommittee of the MAC to structure and monitor the scholars' mentoring and career development and review/approve all scholar research projects. To insure high quality mentoring and adequate oversight of scholars' progress, the Mentoring Committee focused on education for both mentors and scholars, including a clear description and discussion of the expectations for interactions (Blixen, Papp, Hull, Rudick, & Bramstedt, 2007), signed commitments by mentors agreeing to the expectations and the collaborative construction of a detailed, integrated career development plan.

Selection and education of mentors took place between the time applicants to the K12 program successfully competed for a position and actually joined the training program on July first of each year. Selected scholars discussed possible mentors with the MCRTP Co-Director responsible for the mentoring activities. Two mentors were identified for each scholar. The research mentor was in the scholar's intellectual area, responsible for supervising the scholar's research activities and expected to meet with the scholar regularly, usually weekly. A second mentor, a member of the MAC, was responsible for providing career advice and assuring the integration of didactic research and clinical components of the program. The responsibilities and activities of each of the two types of mentors are shown in Table 2.1. Once mentors were agreed upon, they were discussed with the Mentoring Committee. Criteria for approving a mentor included track record in conducting independently funded clinical or translational research, record of successful mentoring, and willingness to comply with the list of mentor responsibilities. If approved, possible mentors were contacted, their responsibilities were outlined, and a preliminary agreement was obtained. After approval of the mentors by the governing committee for the training program, mentors were sent a letter outlining the training, responsibilities, and reimbursement. A signed agreement was obtained from each mentor.

An afternoon of training for mentors occurred prior to the welcoming reception for new scholars each spring. A history of mentoring, stages of mentoring, characteristics of good mentors, and responsibilities of mentees as well as the responsibilities of MCRTP mentors were discussed (Blixen et al., 2007). Mentors received an overview of all aspects of the MCRTP and, beginning in the third year of the program, scholars presented on their mentoring experiences. Mentors were encouraged to ask questions, explore various ways of becoming involved in the program in addition to mentoring, and then to meet the scholars and faculty involved with the program at the reception for new scholars.

CASE STUDY TABLE 2.1
Mentoring Responsibilities in the MCRTP

Responsibilities	Research	MAC
Yearly orientation	√	√
Scholar meetings	Weekly	Every 2 months
Joint career development	√	√
Planned program of study	√	√√
Career development plan	√	√√
Development of research proposal	√√	√
Review of research proposal	√	√
Ensure integration and balance between didactic, research, and clinical components	√	√√
Twice yearly progress reports	√	√
Evaluation activities	√	√

Career Development Plans

Development and Implementation

As mentioned earlier, the Case-Cleveland Clinic MCRTP application proposed a career development plan for each selected scholar. The language in the application describing the plan generally followed the description of a career development plan found in the Mentored Patient-Oriented Research Career Development Award (K23; PA-00-004). Specifically, the Case-Cleveland Clinic MDCRTP application stated:

> A career development plan will be developed by the Clinical Research (CR) Scholar together with the Research and MAC Mentors by the end of the first 6 months of participation in the Program. Less experienced candidates may require a phased developmental period in which the first 1 or 2 year(s) of the award are largely of a didactic nature followed by a period of intense, supervised research experience. Scholars with more experience . . . may need a shorter didactic period . . . The career development plan must be specifically tailored to the needs of the individual CR scholar with the ultimate goal of achieving independence as an effective clinical researcher. The Mentorship Committee will present career development plans for each applicant to the MAC for approval. In consultation with their mentors, CR scholars will prepare a written learning plan that not only identifies key learning objectives, but also means for meeting them as well as a timeline. Each CR scholar will develop, as part of his or her portfolio, individualized targets for each of the elements above (publications; grant submissions; presentations at national meetings) depending on prior experience.

As the Mentorship Committee began to outline the mentoring and career development activities for the MCRTP, it chose to emphasize the Career Development Plans for several reasons. First, based on the considerable experience of the Members of the Mentoring Committee—all senior faculty with successful NIH funding histories—few had planned integrated research, educational, and teaching activities but all recognized the benefit of an integrated plan for career development. Knowing that the goal of the K12 program was to re-engineer the clinical research workforce, the Committee wanted scholars to think carefully about their entire careers rather than focusing only on their research projects. Second, given that the K12 specified multiple mentors and that the Case-Cleveland Clinic MCRTP wanted scholars to benefit from the perspectives of both mentors, focusing on career issues through the development of a plan appeared to be a good vehicle to encourage both mentors to work cooperatively with the scholar. Third, the Committee wanted scholars to observe collegial interchanges and to learn to incorporate different perspectives. It was thought that the Career Development Plans would stimulate role modeling and discussions about critical career decisions. Finally, the Committee wanted scholars to begin early to take responsibility for their own careers.

The Committee believed that the Career Development Plans would foster self-efficacy and provide each of the scholars with easily available benchmarks against which to judge his or her progress.

Career Development Plans are not a new concept; the importance of these plans for fostering self-efficacy is documented in the literature. The business community often uses career growth plans to assist employees in achieving career goals. Documentation suggests that career development plans help individuals to: (1) identify aspirations, interests, strengths, and development opportunities; (2) set realistic expectations for career growth; and (3) develop and implement a plan, and establish follow-up to evaluate progress (Hegstad & Wentling, 2004; Van de Ven, 2007). Bakken and colleagues suggest that it is important to attend to the interaction of personal factors with the research environment and that incorporating and evaluating interventions for self-efficacy could optimize the career development of clinical researchers (Bakken, Byars-Winston, & Wang, 2006). Specifically, they suggest, based on social cognitive career theory, that person-environment interactions from learning experiences promote confidence and that this, in turn, promotes career self-efficacy. The potential value of Career Development Plans rests on the notion of developing self-efficacy, which social cognitive career theory suggests is related to outcome expectations and ultimately career attainment (Gelso & Lent, 2000; Lent & Brown, 1996; Van de Ven, 2007).

There are very recent data to suggest that Career Development Plans do, in actuality, promote career development and may be linked to securing academic positions for post doctoral fellows. As pointed out by Gitlin (2008), Vice Chair of the Board of Directors for the National Postdoctoral Association (NPA), the NPA has focused on ways to assist young scientists develop translational skills including individual development plans (IDPs). IDPs are recommended to promote: (1) self-examination of performance; (2) establishment of medium- and long-term career goals/skills; and (3) development of a timeline with benchmarks to assess progress (Gitlin, 2008). This recommendation is based on the results of a survey, "Doctors without Orders," conducted by Sigma Xi, the Scientific Research Society. Surveying postdoctoral fellows across the United States in 2003 in 46 institutions, including 18 of the top 20 academic centers, this study with 7,600 respondents found that adjusting for sex, citizenship, funding mechanism, field and institution, postdoctoral fellows with the greatest amount of structure and formal training were most satisfied, reported the least conflict, and were more successful in terms of publications. Interestingly, institution features such as good employment benefits and higher salaries were only weakly associated with satisfaction but not associated at all with productivity (Davis, 2005). Focusing on structure, measured in over 24 ways, only one component was associated with all measures of success—a structured plan—including clear responsibilities and performance evaluations (Davis, 2005).

The Mentoring Committee required that a Career Development Plan be developed by each scholar within 6 months of enrollment in the K12 program. The Career Development Plans were to be: (1) developed by the scholar in conjunction with both of his/her mentors; (2) updated yearly; and (3) the Career Development Plan process was to be led by the MAC mentor. Approval of the Career Development Plan by the Mentoring Committee was required for acceptance into the next year of the training program. At the March MAC meeting each year, the Scholar Career Development Plans were presented, and approved, with or without conditions. The suggested content of the Career Development Plan included the following:

Career Goals: Please succinctly describe your career goals for the next 5 years.
Career Objectives: For each goal, please specify two to five objectives that, when met, will result in your achieving your career goal.
Educational Experiences: For each objective, please indicate any educational experiences that will assist you in meeting that objective.
Research Experiences: For each career objective, please indicate any research activities/projects that will assist you in meeting that objective. Please append any research project descriptions and budgets to this document.
Products: For each objective, please indicate what individual products (degrees, publications, presentations, and grants) are expected.
Timeline: Please construct a 2-year timeline displaying the individual objectives, educational activities, research activities, and products.

Further, because the Mentoring Committee wanted the Career Development Plans to be an integrated approach to each scholar's activities, we asked that the plans be displayed as a grid linking educational activities, research projects, products, and deadlines to each goal/objective (Table 2.2).

RESULTS FROM THE INITIAL EXPERIENCE WITH CAREER DEVELOPMENT PLANS. The Career Development Plans were submitted by the end of the first 6 months in the MCRTP. The plans were reviewed by the Mentoring Committee with four approved and recommended to the governing committee of the training program. Four of the Career Development Plans were underdeveloped and were returned to the scholars and mentors with a request to revise and resubmit the Career Development Plan. Problems with the Career Development Plans included vague or overly general goals, lack of integration of educational, research and career-related activities, and a focus solely on research goals without consideration of educational/professional development goals. The four scholars who were asked to

CASE STUDY TABLE 2.2
Career Development Plan

Year 1: July 2006–June 2007

Goal: Become independent researcher studying pediatric sleep and psychosocial trauma

Objectives	Educational/Training Activity	Research Activity	Product/Dates
1. Expand knowledge base about traumatic stress & psychological adjustment of persons exposed to violence and other traumatic events	Course: Developmental psychopathology (Fall 2006) Course: PTSD and traumatic stress (Spring 2007) Ongoing mentoring from scientific mentor	Study on "profiles of adjustment" of children of battered women who participated in CWWV program, using cluster analysis (Fall 2006)	"Profiles" article to be submitted to *Journal of Interpersonal Violence* or *Journal of Family Violence* (Spring 2007)
2. Enhance skill in measurement of psychological trauma	Psychosocial measures of trauma—mentoring from scientific mentor & key psychology faculty Develop reading list of biological markers of trauma Biomarkers training; cortisol & other markers as identified (ongoing)	Study on psychometric properties of DOSE Fall 2006	DOSE psychometric properties poster presented at ISSTS conference (Nov 2006) Biomarkers of trauma reading list completed (Feb 2007) DOSE psychometric properties article submitted (Spring 2007) Consult w/endocrinologist June 2007
3. Enhance skill in measurement of sleep	Mentoring & training in actigraphy from Sleep Medicine group (Fall 2006–Summer 2007)	Study to develop Cleveland Adolescent Sleepiness Questionnaire (CASQ)	CASQ article submitted to SLEEP (Nov 2006) CASQ abstract submitted to APSS review committee (Dec 2006)
4. Advanced training in design, analysis for epidemiologic/clinical studies	No activities year one		

Objectives	Educational/Training Activity	Research Activity	Product/Dates
5. Create a viable research program on effects of violence on children's sleep		Actigraphy feasibility study (Jan–Feb 2007) Develop sleep as mediator study (Spring 2007)	Poster feasibility study-K12 meeting (Spring 2007) Actigraphy feasibility study Submit proposal for "sleep as mediator" pilot study (Aug 2007)
6. Develop leadership & team building skills	CRSP 501 Working in Interdisciplinary Research Teams (Fall 2006)		
7. Hone writing and presentation skills	CRSP 412 Communication in Clinical Research I (Fall 2006) CRSP 413 Communication in Clinical Research II (Spring, 2007) Mentoring by scientific & MAC mentors		Receive feedback on manuscript psychometric properties of DOSE (Fall 2006) Written products under objectives 1–3 Present CASQ results at APSS (June 2007)

Goal: Become effective research team member providing anthropological input on child health/behavioral research

Objectives	Educational/Training Activity	Research Activity	Product/Dates
1. Develop opportunities to collaborate with investigators on local and national levels	Participate in Division's sleep conferences (ongoing) Attend K12 Scholar Seminars (ongoing) Invite anthropology professor to collaborate on children's definition & demarcation of neighborhood (Jan 2007) Participate in Transdisciplinary Research in Energetics & Cancer working group on Psychosocial Determinants of physical activity & eating (ongoing)	Present and participate in Case/VA/Metro Sleep Research Group meeting (Jan 2007) Analyze children's neighborhood boundary data (Spring 2007) Explore opportunities for collaboration with participants in working groups (ongoing)	Chapter on Pediatric sleep apnea Submitted (Nov 2006) Presentation Violence and Sleep in children (Jan 2007) Begin article on children's neighborhood boundaries (Spring 2007)

(Continued)

CASE STUDY TABLE 2.2 (Continued)

Objectives	Educational/Training Activity	Research Activity	Product/Dates
2. Develop opportunity to teach and mentor other investigators and students	Anthropology Guest lecturer—Cross-cultural perspectives on children's sleep (Spring 2007) Continue as ad hoc reviewer for *SLEEP* & *JDBP* (ongoing) UH residents, journal club, leading session on prognosis, May 2007	Provide assistance to: Behav. fellow in analysis of qualitative data pertaining to school bullying (Nov 2006–Spring 2007) Pediatrics asst. professor in using neighborhood level measures (Nov 2006–Spring 2007) Pediatric resident on qualitative methods for studying physicians' coping with the grief process (Nov 2006–ongoing)	Submit article on adolescent perceptions of school bullying (Oct 2007) Complete, "re-usable" PowerPoint presentation on cross-cultural perspectives on children's sleep (Spring 2007)

Year 2: July 2007–June 2008
Goal: Become independent researcher on pediatric sleep and psychosocial trauma

Objectives	Educational/Training Activity	Research Activity	Product/Dates
1. Expand knowledge base about traumatic stress & psychological adjustment of persons exposed to violence and other traumatic events	Continued mentoring from scientific & career mentors		Review article on Effects of Violence on Sleep, including conceptual model (Spring 2008)
2. Enhance skill in measurement of psychological trauma	Continued mentoring on psychosocial measures of trauma—scientific mentor Trauma biomarkers training (ongoing)		Endocrinologist consultation, cortisol July 2007

Objectives	Educational/Training Activity	Research Activity	Product/Dates
3. Enhance skill in measurement of sleep	Continue actigraphy training with sleep medicine group		Actigraphy training completed (Fall 2007)
4. Advanced training in design, implementation, data analysis for epidemiologic/clinical studies	Summer course on mediation analysis with longitudinal data Workshop on longitudinal modeling		
5. Create a viable research program on effects of violence on children's sleep	Continued mentoring from K12 mentors and division chief	Initiate sleep as mediator study	Database preparations completed (December 2007) Research Assistant hired (January 2008) First participants recruited (January 2008)
6. Develop leadership and team building skills	CRSP 502 Leadership CRSP 603 Research Ethics		
7. Hone writing and presentation skills	Continued mentoring from K12 mentors, division chief		Manuscript from objectives above

Goal: Become effective research team member providing anthropological input on child health/behavioral research

Objectives	Educational/Training Activity	Research Activity	Product/Dates
1. Develop opportunities to collaborate with established investigators on local and national levels	Continue participation in: Division's sleep conferences K12 Scholar Seminars Case/VA/Metro Sleep Research Group meeting TREC working group on physical activity, sleep, environment Schubert Center Faculty Associates Working Group	Explore opportunities for collaboration with participants in working groups (ongoing) Assess funding opportunities from govt and foundation sources Collaborate with UAB group on trauma/sleep/health outcomes of women veterans	Submit article on children's neighborhood boundaries to *Am. J. Comm. Psychol.* (Jan 2008) Table of potential foundation supporters to develop grant proposals to cover part of my time as co-PI or collaborating scientist (Jan 2008) Identify specific topics & funding sources (Jan–Feb 2008)

(Continued)

CASE STUDY TABLE 2.2 (Continued)

Objectives	Educational/Training Activity	Research Activity	Product/Dates
			Background lit review for topics (Jan–Feb 2008)
			Develop specific aims/hypotheses (Feb–Apr 2008)
			Complete & submit proposals (Apr 2008–Sep 2008 for initial round)
			Develop other proposals as opportunities emerge (Oct 2008–June 2009)
			Submit background materials, biosketch, etc., to group for inclusion in proposal to Dept. of Defense
2. Develop opportunities to teach & mentor other investigators and students	Develop syllabus for course focused on integration of qualitative and quantitative ("mixed") methods	Serve on Behav. Peds. fellow scholarship oversight committee (ongoing)	Submit article on adolescent perceptions of school bullying (Summer 2007)
	Continue as ad hoc reviewer for *SLEEP* & *JDBP*	Judicious selection of other opportunities as they appear	Mixed methods syllabus (Spring 2008)
			Complete analysis of study of SDB & depression in obese children
			Develop other products (manuscripts, presentations) as opportunities arise

revise and resubmit their Career Development Plans had their plans approved on the second submission.

The scholars' reactions were solicited during a seminar discussion and were positive but reflected the challenges that developing a Career Development Plan posed. They all said that "developing a career plan was much harder than expected" and that it was the first time that they had been asked to think broadly about their careers rather than focusing on a single research project. They called it "an important learning experience that helped broaden their perspectives and products." The link across education, research and career development activities, as well as over the 2-year time period, helped each scholar to develop a personal roadmap. Many scholars commented that the Career Development Plan would serve as a way for them and their mentors to judge their progress, and the plans would serve as guides for making career choices. As one scholar said, "If I'm asked to do something that has absolutely nothing to do with any of my objectives, I now know that I need to think twice about it."

In the experience of a co-author James Spilsbury, who was a scholar and whose Career Development Plan appears in Table 2.2, one critical characteristic of the Career Development Plan is that it is a "living" document that can be modified over time to include new, advantageous research and educational opportunities that arise, provided these opportunities fit with overall career goals and objectives. Moreover, the Career Development Plan can become increasingly more detailed to provide guidance as needed (e.g., adding benchmarks and deadlines for a developing and submitting a proposal to a specific funding agency or foundation). An additional advantage of the Career Development Plan is that it encourages thinking about how to develop career-enhancing products from research and educational activities whenever possible. For example, in the case of the Career Development Plan presented here, the "term paper" requirement for the course on developmental psychopathology was met by analyzing an existing dataset and writing up the results as a manuscript for publication in a peer-review journal (Spilsbury et al., 2008). However, developing a useful Career Development Plan takes considerable reflection and time; it is not the type of document that can be written in a single, short sitting.

Although the Career Development Plans were not specifically evaluated, the evaluations of mentoring for the MCRTP were quite positive. In year 2 of the program, scholars ($n = 16$) active in the program were asked to complete the Mentorship Profile Questionnaire and the Mentorship Effectiveness Scale (Berk et al., 2005). Scholars completed these online, confidential questionnaires between April and May 2008. In all, 14 of 16 scholars (88%) completed both surveys on one or both of their mentors. Results are reported in Table 2.3. Results indicate overall high satisfaction with the mentoring relationship where in 62% of cases, scholars

CASE STUDY TABLE 2.3

Case-Cleveland Clinic Multidisciplinary Clinical Research Training Program (MCRTP) Scholars' Perceptions of Their Mentoring Relationships

Questions	N	%
What is the role of your mentor? (Check all that apply)		
Teacher	15	57.69
Counselor	13	50.00
Advisor	24	92.31
Sponsor	5	19.23
Advocate	19	73.08
Resource	19	73.08
Other, please specify	3	11.54
How often, in the past 6 months, did you communicate? (e.g., e-mail, in person, telephone)		
Daily	5	19.2
Once a week	9	34.6
Once a month	5	19.2
Once every other month	3	11.5
Less than every other month	1	3.9
Other, please specify	3	11.5
Who was most likely to initiate the communication? (Check only one)		
The mentor	0	0.0
I, the mentee	10	38.5
Both were equally likely to initiate communication	16	61.5
Please check all of the following that resulted from your interaction with your mentor and specify or describe below		
Publication	15	57.7
Presentation or poster	17	65.4
New teaching method or strategy	8	30.8
Clinical expertise	4	15.4
Conducting research	20	76.9
Service activities (e.g., community service, professional organization)	6	23.1
Development of a program	6	23.1
Job change or promotion	5	19.2
Grant writing/grant submission	20	76.9
Educational opportunities (e.g., participated in a course or program)	13	50.0
Other, please specify	4	15.4

Questions	N	%
Indicate the extent to which you agree or disagree with each statement listed below. My mentor:		
Was accessible		
Agree	7	26.9
Strongly agree	17	65.4
Demonstrated professional integrity		
Agree	4	15.4
Strongly agree	21	80.8
Demonstrated content-specific expertise in my area of need		
Agree	5	19.2
Strongly agree	16	61.5
Was approachable		
Agree	5	19.2
Strongly agree	21	80.8
Was supportive and encouraging		
Agree	2	7.7
Strongly agree	23	88.5
Provided constructive and useful critiques of my work		
Agree	6	23.1
Strongly agree	19	73.1
Motivated me to improve my work product		
Agree	7	26.9
Strongly agree	18	69.2
Was helpful in providing direction and guidance on professional issues (e.g., networking)		
Agree	5	19.2
Strongly agree	20	76.9
Answered my questions satisfactorily (e.g., timely response, clear, comprehensive)		
Agree	7	28.0
Strongly agree	17	68.0
Acknowledged my contributions appropriately (e.g., committee contributions, awards)		
Agree	5	19.2
Strongly agree	14	53.9
Suggested appropriate resources (e.g., experts, electronic contacts, source materials)		
Agree	5	19.2
Strongly agree	19	73.1
Challenged me to extend my abilities (e.g., risk-taking, try a new professional activity, draft a section of an article)		
Agree	6	24.0
Strongly agree	16	64.0

responded that both the mentor and the scholar were equally likely to initiate communication. The relationships were highly productive; scholars responded that interactions with mentor(s) resulted in the following outcomes: conduct of clinical research (n = 20 [77%]); grant writing; grant submission (n = 20 [77%]); presentation or poster (n = 17 [65%]); and publication (n = 15 [58%]).

CONCLUSION

Career Development Plans provided an excellent opportunity to focus attention on scholars' careers rather than specific research projects, served as a vehicle for involving mentors in their scholars' development, stimulated lively collegial exchanges, and provided scholars with a tool to benchmark their progress as well as determine the appropriateness of additional educational and research opportunities. The Career Development Plan proved to be an effective means to promote mentoring across multiple disciplines and institutions.

Additionally, the emphasis on mentoring in the MCRTP resulted in a number of important lessons. First, creating a culture-valuing mentoring was critical. Offering training, a small financial incentive, and public recognition for outstanding mentoring produced mentoring relationships that worked. Second, establishing expectations for both scholars and mentors proved invaluable and insured that beneficial interactions occurred. Finally, a procedure for resolving misunderstandings and working with scholars to assist them in establishing solid relationships with their mentors who met their needs fostered productive, positive interactions.

REFERENCES

Bakken, L. L., Byars-Winston, A., Wang, M. F. (2006). Viewing clinical research career development through the lens of social cognitive career theory. *Advances in Health Sciences Education, 11*(1), 91–110.

Berk, R. A., Berg, J., Mortimer, R., Walton-Moss, B., & Yeo, T. P. (2005). Measuring the effectiveness of faculty mentoring relationships. *Academic Medicine, 80*(1), 66–71.

Blixen, C. E., Papp, K. K., Hull, A. L., Rudick, R. A., & Bramstedt, K. A. (2007). Developing a mentorship program for clinical researchers. *Journal of Continuing Education in Health Prof*essions, 27(2), 86–93.

Boyle, P., & Boice, B. (1998). Systematic mentoring for new faculty teachers and graduate teaching assistants. *Innovative Higher Education, 22*(3), 157–179.

Cupples, S. A. (1999). Selection, care, and feeding of a research mentor. *Alzheimer Disease & Associated Disorders, 13*(Suppl. 1), S22–S28.

Davis, G. (2005). Doctors without orders. *American Scientist, 93*(3, Suppl.), 1–13.

Erdem, F., & Aytemur, J. (2008). Mentoring—A relationship based on trust: Qualitative research. *Public Personnel Management, 37*(1), 55–65.

Garman, K. A., Wingard, D. L., & Reznik, V. (2001). Development of junior faculty's self-efficacy: Outcomes of a National Center of Leadership in Academic Medicine. *Academic Medicine, 76*(10, Suppl.), S74–S76.

Gelso, C. J., & Lent, R. W. (2000). Scientific training and scholarly productivity: The person, the training environment, and their interaction. In S. D. Brown & R. W. Lent (Eds.), *Handbook of counseling psychology* (3rd ed., pp. 109–139). New York: Wiley.

Gitlin, J. (2008). Establishing career platforms for postdocs through individual development plans. *Disease Models & Mechanisms, 1*(1), 15.

Goldstein, J. L., & Brown, M. S. (1997). The clinical investigator: Bewitched, bothered, and bewildered—But still beloved. *Journal of Clinical Investigation, 99*(12), 2803–2812.

Hegstad, C. D., & Wentling, R. M. (2004). The development and maintenance of exemplary formal mentoring programs in Fortune 500 companies. *Human Resource Development Quarterly, 15*(4), 421–448.

James, S. P. (2003). This month at the NIH: NIH roadmap: Accelerating medical discovery to improve health. *Gastroenterology, 125*(6), 1573.

Lent, R. W., & Brown, S. D. (1996). Social cognitive approach to career development: An overview. *Career Development Quarterly, 44*(4), 310–321.

Levinson, D. J., Darrow, C. N., Klein, E. G., Levinson, M. H., & McKee, B. (1978). *Seasons of a man's life.* New York: Knopf.

Ludwig, S., & Stein, R. E. (2008). Anatomy of mentoring. *Journal of Pediatrics, 152*(2), 151–152.

McLellan, F. (2003). NIH director reviews first year on the job. "Roadmap" calls for reorganisation of basic and clinical research. *Lancet, 362*(9381), 381–382.

Nathan, D. G. (1998). Clinical research: Perceptions, reality, and proposed solutions. National Institutes of Health Director's Panel on Clinical Research. *Journal of the American Medical Association, 280*(16), 1427–1431.

Nathan, D. G., & Wilson, J. D. (2003). Clinical research and the NIH—A report card. *New England Journal of Medicine, 349*(19), 1860–1865.

Rogers, J., Monteiro, F. M., & Nora, A. (2008). Toward measuring the domains of mentoring. *Family Medicine, 40*(4), 259–263.

Sands, R. G., Parson, L. A., & Duane, J. (1991). Faculty mentoring faculty in a public university. *Journal of Higher Education, 62*(2), 174–193.

Sambunjak, D., Straus, S. E., & Marusić, A. (2006). Mentoring in academic medicine: A systematic review. *Journal of the American Medical Association, 296*(9), 1103–1115.

Spilsbury, J. C., Kahana, S., Drotar, D., Creeden, R., Flannery, D., & Friedman, S. (2008). Profiles of behavioral problems in children who witness domestic violence. *Violence and Victims, 23*(1), 3–17.

Van de Ven, F. (2007). Fulfilling the promise of career development: Getting to the "heart" of the matter. *Organizational Development Journal, 25*(3), 45–50.

Wang, L. (2003). 'Roadmap' gives new direction to trans-NIH research. *Journal of the National Cancer Institute, 95*(23), 1741.

Wasserstein, A. G., Quistberg, D. A., & Shea, J. A. (2007). Mentoring at the University of Pennsylvania: Results of a faculty survey. *Journal of General Internal Medicine, 22*(2), 210–214.

Webster's Ninth New Collegiate Dictionary. (1983). Springfield, MA: Merriam-Webster.

Zerhouni, E. (2003). Medicine. The NIH Roadmap. *Science, 302*(5642), 63–72.

THREE

Mentoring Students
and Junior Professionals

Research suggests that students at all levels of their training value mentorship. Student nurses participating in a study of mentoring indicated that mentors play a significant role in clinical learning (Earnshaw, 1995). Surveys of medical school students indicate that approximately 90% of those surveyed rate mentorship as either important or very important or are interested in developing a mentoring relationship (Aagaard & Hauer, 2003; Ricer, Fox, & Miller, 1995). Similarly, surveys of participants in medical residency training programs have found that most participants believe that mentoring is important during this phase of their training (Ramanan, Taylor, Davis, & Phillips, 2006).

It is not possible within a single volume to discuss all issues relevant to mentoring across all health careers. Accordingly, this chapter focuses on mentoring high school and undergraduate students who may be interested in pursuing a career in a health-related field; nursing students and junior nurses; medical students, residents, and fellows; and graduate students in other health-related fields. Case Study 3 authored by Clegg and colleagues that follows this chapter provides a more detailed view of mentoring medical residents in the field of psychiatry.

MENTORING HIGH SCHOOL STUDENTS
AND UNDERGRADUATES FOR HEALTH-RELATED CAREERS

Mentorship at the high school and undergraduate levels is decidedly less common than at the graduate level. One study of undergraduate students at a west coast university found that 67% of the respondents had experienced difficulty in identifying a mentor during the previous year (Jacobi, 1989). These difficulties may be intensified for women and minority students (Johnson, 1989). The relative scarcity of mentoring at the undergraduate level may be due, in part, to time limitations and students' need to acquire a foundation across a range of arts and sciences (Byrne & Keefe, 2002).

The role of the mentor at the high school and undergraduate levels has often consisted of the mentor's provision to the mentee of advice regarding possible career options, sources of recommendation letters, and the packaging of applications for admission to the graduate programs of interest (Johnson, Settimi, & Rogers, 2001). However, significantly more may be required if younger students are to be successful in their pursuit of a career in the health professions. In contrast to this limited view of mentors' functions, effective mentoring at the undergraduate level that encompasses the provision of information, guidance, advice, encouragement, support, sponsorship, and acceptance, and serving as role model, has been found to be associated with academic success (Astin, 1977; Pascarella & Terenzini, 1977; Tracey & Sedlacek, 1985; Wilson, Gaff, Dienst, Wood, & Bavry, 1975).

A variety of innovative programs have been developed to foster the interest of high school students in a health-related career. As one example, the Howard Hughes Medical Institute has provided the State of Maryland's Montgomery County Schools with a grant that allows high school students and their teachers to interact with NIH scientists who serve as mentors (Delgado, 2006). The National Heart, Lung, and Blood Institute (NHBLI) has developed a program that requires its funded investigators to participate in science training and provide mentoring to help develop a pool of students who are interested in pursuing careers in scientific research (Tomanek et al., 2005). It has also been suggested that undergraduate students should be exposed to research during their undergraduate years in college and throughout their student careers in medical school for those who pursue a career in medicine (McPhaul, 2004).

Programs also exist at the undergraduate level that encourage students to explore and pursue scientific research. One undergraduate honors program at the University of Hawaii provided minority students with mentoring over a 2-year period, during which they completed and presented their research projects (Inouye, 1995). The University of Maryland developed a bridge program for undergraduate students from underrepresented groups that fostered collaborations with research faculty (Perry, 1997).

It has been suggested that undergraduates may not receive realistic advice regarding the likelihood of their admission to medical school, and that they may actually be shortchanged by advisers who fail to apprise them of the many career options available to them in the various health professions (Johnson, Settimi, & Rogers, 2001). These alternative options include careers in social work, occupational therapy, respiratory therapy, physical therapy, dance and music therapy, public health, and others.

MENTORING STUDENTS AND JUNIOR PROFESSIONALS
IN NONMEDICAL CLINICAL CAREERS

Significant research has been conducted in the field of nursing that is potentially relevant to other clinical disciplines, such as social work, psychology, physical therapy, occupational therapy, and others. Professionals in each of these fields may experience high levels of stress due to the nature of their work, undergo transitions during their professional careers, and expend considerable energy through emotional labor. This portion of the chapter draws on the nursing and other literature that pertains to these issues and that may be useful to readers across a variety of clinical disciplines.

Like nursing students and more junior nurses (Hyland, Miller, & Parker, 1988), individuals training in other clinical professions may experience high levels of stress, particularly in the context of unfamiliar clinical situations in which they bear significant responsibility for others' well-being (Hyland, Millar, & Parker, 1988). Unlike the classroom environment, which is limited for the most part to exchanges between students and faculty, the clinical environment demands familiarity with and an ability to interact with staff members, patients, patients' family members, and unexpected occurrences (Cahill, 1996; Papp, Markkanen, & von Bonsdorff, 2003) and, in some situations, manage equipment. Accordingly, successful mentoring requires that the mentor and mentee be cognizant of the developmental process through which students will acquire greater familiarity with, knowledge of, and confidence in clinical settings.

Research suggests that nurses entering the profession develop along a four-stage trajectory. Although the process delineated here has been applied to nurses, clinicians in other fields may evolve professionally along a somewhat similar trajectory. The first stage, that of the apprenticeship, is characterized by dependency on the mentor and a requirement for close supervision (Myers Schim, 1990). It may be particularly important during this early career period to assist students and junior professionals to understand the application of theory to practice (Wilson-Barnett et al., 1995). During the second stage, the relationship between the mentor and the mentee becomes more collegial and requires less supervision (Myers Schim, 1990). During the third stage, individuals may take on the role of mentoring others junior to themselves. The fourth stage is characterized by the assumption of increased levels of responsibility for both personnel and patients. Mentoring may be particularly important for those who wish to move through this career trajectory (Woolnough, Davidson, & Fielden, 2006). In addition, during each stage of professional development, the mentor should ideally address with the mentee issues that arise in seven categories of needs: psychological, belonging, esteem, cognitive, aesthetic, and self-actualization (Williams & McLean, 1992).

Not surprisingly, then, mentoring has been found to be particularly critical during periods of professional transition (Andersen, 1990; Cahill, 1996; Earnshaw, 1995; Phillips, Davies, & Neary, 1996a, 1996b; Smith & Gray, 2001), when individuals may be less certain of their knowledge and less secure in their role (Bradby, 1990; Brown & Olshansky, 1997; Kelly & Matthews, 2001). Nursing students transitioning into actual practice have described feeling lost, bewildered, and overwhelmed (Bradby, 1990, p. 1222). Even transitions into a different practice situation may create new stresses and uncertainties (Dean, 1998; Houghton, 2003; McNamara, Wadell, & Colvin, 1995; Rasmussen, Norberg, & Sandman, 1995; Rasmussen, Sandman, & Norberg, 1997; Rosser & King, 2003; Suen & Chow, 2001).

The concept of emotional labor refers to the requirement that the individual suppress feeling to maintain an outward appearance, through face-to-face contact, that suggests to others that they are cared for in a safe place (Hochschild, 1983). Emotional labor has traditionally been associated with professions in which women predominate and, as such, has often been undervalued (James, 1993). Nevertheless, the concept may be relevant to men in the clinical professions as well. A mentor can help the clinical student or junior professional to examine the benefits and difficulties of emotional contact with patients and provide assistance and support, as the student or junior professional identifies strategies to deal with the range of emotions that he or she is experiencing (Smith & Gray, 2001). This support may be particularly critical for the mentee during periods of transition, when the mentee's level of stress may be intensified.

It has been suggested that mentoring relationships premised on social learning theory (Bandura, 1977) may be particularly helpful during transition periods (Masny, Ropka, Peterson, Fetzer, & Daly, 2008). According to social learning theory, individuals develop the ability to perform a skill by learning the behavior, seeing the behavior, receiving feedback on their own performance of the behavior, and developing a sense of self-efficacy in performing that behavior. Mentoring using this approach may help to reinforce and enhance junior clinicians' practice skills in new environments (Masny et al., 2008).

Questions have been raised as to whether students in clinical professions are best mentored by those who are closer to them on the career hierarchy in that field or by one or more individuals in an allied clinical field (Earnshaw, 1995; Gibson & Heartfield, 2005). Each approach offers distinct advantages. A mentor in the same profession, particularly one who is close to the mentee's level of expertise, may be more understanding of the mentee's situation because he or she shares somewhat similar training and professional experiences. However, the identification of a suitable mentor in an allied field may more easily facilitate the expansion of the mentee's professional network (Hutchings, Williamson, & Humphreys, 2005; Mitchell, 2003).

Whether the mentor should be involved in the formal assessment of the student's or junior professional's performance has been the focus of some debate. Various authors have suggested that the formal assessment is a critical component of mentoring functions (Morris, John, & Keen, 1988), whereas others have argued that the mentor's fulfillment of a formal assessment function would conflict with his or her nurturing role (Anforth, 1992; Burnard, 1989; Hyde, 1988).

MENTORING STUDENTS, RESIDENTS, AND FELLOWS IN MEDICINE

Mentoring during all phases of medical training is important to individuals in their acquisition of the necessary skills and knowledge. Medical students at the earliest stages of their training may benefit from more directive mentoring that focuses on skill development and includes positive and constructive feedback (Rose, Rukstalis, & Schuckit, 2005). Areas of mentoring that have been identified by residents as most critical include career planning and the conduct of research, which may be most easily addressed if mentors and mentees are matched based on their specialty/subspecialty or research interests (Quaas, Berkowitz, & Tracy, 2009). However, once the student has developed the necessary skills, the mentor's role may become more like that of a consultant.

Mentoring may also support the efforts of medical school students and junior physicians to assimilate as professionals in their communities (Garmel, 2004; Rogstad & Talbot, 2001; Steiner, Pathman, Jones, Williams, & Riggins, 1999) and help to foster a sense of professionalism and professional behavior among new physicians (Larkin, 2003; Reynolds, 1994). Professionally desirable behaviors, such as protecting a patient's interests and confidentiality, participating in the teaching of other students and staff, discussing difficult issues with patients and their families with compassion, are to be valued in themselves but also go a long way toward avoiding later litigation by aggrieved families (Larkin, 1999, 2003). Role modeling of these desired behaviors by mentors may be particularly critical to their development by medical students and new physicians (Kenny, Mann, & MacLeod, 2003). Despite the importance of modeling such behaviors, several studies suggest that medical faculty are frequently poor role models for physician–patient relationships (Beaudoin et al., 1998; Maheux et al., 2000).

Mentoring students at all levels of their medical training may be important to reduce the stress and burnout that is often experienced (Collier, McCue, Markus, & Smith, 2002; Shanafelt, Bradley, Wipf, & Back, 2002), which may result from a lack of autonomy, work overload, role conflict, and excessive paperwork (Cordes, & Dougherty, 1993; Hirsch, 1999; Ramirez, Graham, Richards, Cull, & Gregory, 1996). Burnout, defined as a syndrome characterized by emotional exhaustion, negative and cynical thoughts toward other people, and a reduced sense of personal accomplishment (Maslach & Jackson, 1986), is of concern because of its correlation with psychological disturbance (Ramirez et al., 1996), anxiety, and depression (Hirsch, 1999), and its potential impact on the quality of patient care (Hirsch, 1999; Linzer et al., 2001).

These feelings may be particularly acute among women and minorities. Research indicates that, compared with men, women are more likely to experience feelings of depression during the first year of medical school (Parkerson, Broadhead, & Tse, 1990), are more likely to experience role strain, and are more likely to seek psychiatric help (Dickstein, Stephenson, & Hinz, 1990). Black and Hispanic medical students are also more likely to experience feelings of distress compared with their non-Hispanic White counterparts (Pyskoty, Richman, & Flaherty, 1990). (Whether female, Black, and Hispanic students actually experience higher levels of stress or are more open and/or honest in reporting it is unclear from the literature.) Studies continue to suggest that, despite the recognition of the importance of a mentoring relationship during professional training, women and underrepresented minorities at all levels of training are less likely to have access to a mentoring relationship (Bogart & Redner, 1985; Lewis, 2003; Ramanan et al., 2006; Sirridge, 1985; See also Chapter 4) and are less likely to receive adequate mentoring when mentoring is available (Ramanan et al., 2006; See also Chapter 4). As a result, peer groups may be necessary to provide support in addressing issues related to gender, race, and ethnicity (Hilberman et al., 1975; Weston & Paterson, 1980).

Despite the recognized importance of a mentor during all phases of medical training, approximately two-thirds of medical school students (Aagaard & Hauer, 2003) and one-half of interns and residents (Ramanan et al., 2006) report that they did not have a mentor. Significant barriers reduce the likelihood that a student will have a mentoring relationship. These include limited contact with professors (Igartua, 1997; Reynolds, 1994; Ricer et al., 1995), student discomfort asking for mentoring, and students' failure to meet anyone with similar interests (Aagaard & Hauer, 2003). Students may also refrain from seeking out a mentor because of their immediate focus on "getting through" (Flach, Smith, Smith, & Glasser, 1982). Medical school students may subscribe to the "doctor–patient" model of mentoring, in that they believe that mentoring is only for those students who are in trouble, and the search for a mentor implies that there is something wrong (Flach et al., 1982; Taylor, 1980). Increased clinical, research, and administrative demands on medical school faculty (Levy et al., 2004) and the faculty reward system at many medical schools that emphasizes research and publication (Angell, 1986; Petersdorf, 1986) and fails to reward teaching and mentoring may cause faculty to view mentoring as a burden and discourage senior faculty from undertaking mentoring functions (Reynolds, 1994; Quaas et al., 2009; cf. Larkin, 2003). As a result, medical school students are more likely to develop relationships with attendings and residents than with faculty members (Cochran, Paukert, Scales, & Neumayer, 2004; Tekian, Jalovecky, & Hruska, 2001).

MENTORING MASTER'S AND DOCTORAL STUDENTS

Despite the widespread support for mentoring relationships for graduate students, a large proportion of graduate students in the health professions and sciences lack a mentor. For example, approximately one-third to one-half of graduate students and interns in psychology do not have a mentor (Atkinson, Casas, & Neville, 1994; Clark, Harden, & Johnson, 2000; Cronan-Hillix, Gensheimer, Cronan-Hillix, & Davidson, 1986; Kirchner, 1969; Mintz, Bartels, & Rideout, 1995). The lack of mentorship may be due, at least in part, to the lack of recognition or reward for faculty who do mentor students and the disproportionate demands often placed on female faculty to provide mentoring (Dickinson & Johnson, 2000). In many cases, graduate students must initiate the mentoring relationship themselves (Clark et al., 2000), a task that many students find difficult (Waldeck, Orrego, Plax, & Kearney, 1997) and that places those students who are less assertive at a disadvantage (Clark et al., 2000). Students searching for a mentor commonly employ one or more of a variety of strategies, including prearranging a working relationship with the targeted faculty mentor, enrolling in a specific course to ensure frequent contact, searching for a faculty member with similar interest, seeking counsel from the potential faculty member, and/or periodically providing teaching assistance (Waldeck et al., 1997).

Relatively few studies have attempted to examine the direct effects of mentoring on student productivity or commitment. Green and Bauer (1995) found from their 2-year study of 233 entering PhD students that after controlling for students' baseline characteristics, such as ability and level of commitment, the psychosocial, career, and collaboration functions of mentoring were unrelated to student productivity. However, students' baseline characteristics, such as their prior research experience, were directly related to the production of a greater number of publications and paper submissions. The researchers also found that students with greater quantitative aptitude, prior research experience, and a targeted (preselected) mentor were more likely to have collaborations with their mentor. In contrast to these findings, Paglis, Green and Bauer (2006) found from their 5½-year longitudinal study of PhD students drawn from 24 academic departments of "hard" sciences that mentoring was significantly associated with mentee productivity and self-efficacy, even after controlling for ability and attitudes at the time of their entry into the PhD program. No association was found, however, between mentoring and level of commitment to a research career.

The current economic climate may well have increased the complexities of mentoring doctoral students in the health-related professions with respect to their career plans. PhD students aspiring to full-time tenured academic positions may find it difficult to achieve that goal. As of 1997, 43% of instructional faculty and staff in U.S. colleges and universities were employed on a part-time basis (Anon., 2000). Almost two-thirds of individuals granted PhD degrees in the life sciences during 1963–1964 held tenure-track appointments 10 years later; that figure had decreased to 38% among those granted PhD degrees during 1985–1986. The proportion of individuals who had PhDs in the life sciences and held "permanent" positions in industry, academia, or government declined from 87% in 1975 to 73% in 1995 (Tilghman, 1998).

Additionally, doctoral training in general has been criticized for its failure to adequately prepare doctoral students to meet the challenges of today's job markets. Although the current technological and economic demands of the job market require individuals to make connections between and across diverse disciplines, many doctoral programs continue to be narrowly focused and actually discourage interdisciplinarity (Nyquist, 2002). This suggests that doctoral students in health-related professions would be best served by having multiple mentors with a variety of skills and perspectives rather than mentorship based on the traditional dyadic model.

Many universities have developed extensive guides to assist both faculty and graduate students in their respective roles as mentors and mentees (Case Western Reserve University, 2007; University of Michigan, 2006; University of Nebraska—Lincoln, 2009; University of Washington, 2005a, 2005b). The depth of that advice, and the extent to which it builds on professional literature relating to mentoring, varies across institutions. Although not career specific, much of the advice is relevant to graduate students in the health professions, such as social work, psychology, and the basic sciences.

SUMMARY

Published literature suggests that it is relatively rare for high school students and undergraduates to enjoy what might be considered a mentoring relationship, in contrast to a relationship focused solely on short-term career advice, for example, choice of college or graduate school, selection of a major, and so on. The occurrence of mentoring relationships at these levels appears to be serendipitous. However, the projected shortage of professionals in health-related careers, including nursing, medicine, and ancillary health professions and the apparent benefits of mentoring argue for the planned establishment of mentoring relationships for high school and undergraduate students who show interest and/or promise in pursuing health-related careers.

The barriers to the formation of mentoring relationships in graduate and professional schools follow common themes: lack of faculty time, lack of reward or support for faculty who serve as mentors, faculty burnout, and inadequate contact with faculty. Responsibility for these impediments cannot be attributed to faculty alone but must also be placed on the currently existing systems and infrastructures that have erected these barriers. Nevertheless, with the exception of some exemplary programs, it is the faculties and administrations that have established and now perpetuate those systems that appear unable and/or unwilling to provide sufficient resources to mentoring functions. It is the faculties and administrations that can ultimately choose to realign priorities to facilitate the establishment of effective mentoring programs and relationships. These organizational and programmatic issues are addressed in Chapter 5.

REFERENCES

Aagaard, E. M., & Hauer, K. E. (2003). A cross-sectional descriptive study of mentoring relationships formed by medical students. *Journal of General Internal Medicine, 18*, 298–302.

Andersen, S. L. (1991). Preceptor teaching strategies: Behaviours that facilitate role transition in senior nursing students. *Journal of Nursing Staff Development, 7*(4), 171–175.

Anforth, P. (1992). Mentors, not assessors. *Nurse Education Today, 12*, 299–302.

Angell, M. (1986). Publish or perish: A proposal. *Annals of Internal Medicine, 104*, 261–262.

Anon. (2000). The nation: Faculty and staff. *Chronicle of Higher Education 2000–2001 Almanac Issue*, 38.

Astin, A. W. (1977). *Four critical years: Effects of college on beliefs, attitudes, and knowledge.* San Francisco: Jossey-Bass.

Atkinson, D. R., Casas, A., & Neville, H. (1994). Ethnic minority psychologists: Whom they mentor and benefits they derive from the process. *Journal of Multicultural Counseling and Development, 22*, 37–48.

Bandura, A. (1977). *Social learning theory.* Englewood Cliffs, NJ: Prentice-Hall.

Beaudoin, C., Maheux, B., Cote, L., Des Marchais, J. E., Jean, P., & Berkson, L. (1998). Clinical teachers as humanistic caregivers and educators: Perceptions of senior clerks and second-year residents. *Canadian Medical Association Journal, 159*, 765–769.

Bogart, G. A., & Redner, R. L. (1985). How mentoring affects the professional development of women in psychology. *Research and Practice, 16*, 851–859.

Bradby, M. (1990). Status passage into nursing: Another view of the process of socialization into nursing. *Journal of Advanced Nursing, 15*, 1220–1225.

Brown, M., & Olshansky, E. F. (1997). From limbo to legitimacy: A theoretical model of the transition to the primary nurse practitioner role. *Nursing Research, 46*, 46–51.

Burnard, P. (1989). The role of mentor. *Journal of District Nursing, 8*(3), 8–17.

Byrne, M. W., & Keefe, M. R. (2002). Building research competence in nursing through mentoring. *Journal of Nursing Scholarship, 34*(4), 391–396.

Cahill, H. (1996). A qualitative analysis of student nurses' experiences of mentorship. *Journal of Advanced Nursing, 24*, 791–799.

Case Western Reserve University. (2007). *A mentoring guidebook for faculty: Helping graduate students grown into respected professionals and trusted colleagues.* Cleveland, OH: Graduate Student Senate of Case Western Reserve University.

Clark, R. A., Harden, S. L., & Johnson, W. B. (2000). Mentor relationships in clinical psychology doctoral training: Results of a national survey. *Teaching of Psychology, 27*(4), 262–268.

Cochran, A., Paukert, J. L., Sacles, E. M., & Neumayer, L. A. (2004). How medical students define surgical mentors. *American Journal of Surgery, 187*, 698–701.

Collier, V. U., McCue, J. D., Markus, A., & Smith, L. (2002). Stress in medical residency: Status quo after a decade of reform? *Annals of Internal Medicine, 136*, 384–390.

Cordes, C. L., & Dougherty, T. W. (1993). A review and integration of research on job burnout. *Academy of Management Review, 18*, 621–656.

Cronan-Hillix, T., Gensheimer, L. K., Cronan-Hillix, W. A., & Davidson, W. S. (1986). Students' views of mentors in psychology graduate training. *Teaching of Psychology, 13*, 123–127.

Dean, R. A. (1998). Occupational stress in hospice care: Causes and coping strategies. *The American Journal of Hospice and Palliative Care, 15*(3), 151–154.

Delgado, C. (2006). NIH high school protégés honored. *NIH Record, 58*(13), 8–9.

Dickinson, S. C., & Johnson, W. B. (2000). Mentoring in clinical psychology doctoral programs: A national survey of directors of training. *The Clinical Supervisor, 19*(1), 137–152.

Dickstein, L. J., Stephenson, M. S., & Hinz, L. D. (1990). Psychiatric impairment in medical students. *Academic Medicine, 65*, 588–592.

Earnshaw, G. J. (1995). Mentorship: The students' views. *Nurse Education Today, 15*, 274–279.

Flach, D. H., Smith, M. F., Smith, W. G., & Glasser, M. L. (1982). Faculty mentors for medical students. *Journal of Medical Education, 57*, 514–520.

Garmel, G. M. (2004). Mentoring medical students in academic emergency medicine. *Academic Emergency Medicine, 11*, 1351–1357.

Gibson, T., & Heartfield, M. (2005). Mentoring for nurses in general practice: An Australian study. *Journal of Interprofessional Care, 19*(1), 50–62.

Green, S. G., & Bauer, T. N. (1995). Supervisory mentoring by advisers: Relationships with doctoral student potential, productivity, and commitment. *Personnel Psychology, 48*, 537–561.

Hilberman, E., Konanc, J., Perez-Reyes, M., Hunter, R., Scagnelli, J., & Sanders, S. (1975). Support groups for women in medical school: A first-year program. *Journal of Medical Education, 50*, 867–875.

Hirsch, G. (1999). Physician career management: Organizational strategies for the 21st century. *Physician Executive, 25*, 30–36.

Hochschild, A. (1983). *The managed heart.* Berkeley, CA: University of California Press.

Houghton, C. (2003). A mentoring program for school nurses. *The Journal of School Nursing, 19*(1), 24–29.

Hutchings, A., Williamson, G., & Humphreys, A. (2005). Supporting learners in clinical practice: Capacity issues. *Journal of Clinical Nursing, 14*, 945–955.

Hyde, J. (1988). Lean on me. *Nursing Standard, 3*, 22–24.

Hyland, M. E., Millar, J., & Parker, S. (1988). How hospital ward nurses treat learner nurses. *Journal of Advanced Nursing, 13*, 472–477.

Igartua, K. (1997). Fostering faculty mentorship of junior medical students [letter]. *Academic Medicine, 72*, 3.

Inouye, J. (1995). A research development program for minority honors students. *Journal of Nursing Education, 34*(6), 268–271.

Jacobi, M. (1989). *Student services assessment: Report on undergraduate student problems.* Los Angeles: University of California.

Jacobi, M. (1991). Mentoring and undergraduate academic success: A literature review. *Review of Educational Research, 61*, 505–532.

James, N. (1993). Divisions of emotional labour: Disclosure and cancer. In S. Fineman (Ed.), *Emotions in organizations* (pp. 94–117). London: Sage.

Johnson, C. S. (1989). Mentoring programs. In M. L. Upcraft & J. Gardner (Eds.), *The freshman year experience: Helping students survive and succeed in college* (pp. 118–128). San Francisco: Jossey-Bass.

Johnson, T. R. B., Settimi, P. D., & Rogers, J. L. (2001). Mentoring for the health professions. *New Directions for Teaching and Learning, 85*, 25–34.

Kelly, N. R., & Matthews, M. (2001). The transition to first position as nurse practitioner. *Journal of Nurse Education, 40*, 156–162.

Kenny, N. P., Mann, K. V., & MacLeod, H. (2003). Role modeling in physicians' professional formation: Reconsidering an essential but untapped educational strategy. *Academic Medicine, 78*(12), 1203–1210.

Kirchner, E. P. (1969). Graduate education in psychology: Retrospective views of advanced degree recipients. *Journal of Clinical Psychology, 25*, 207–213.

Larkin, G. L. (1999). Evaluating professionalism in emergency medicine: Clinical ethical competence. *Academic Emergency Medicine, 6*, 302–311.

Larkin, G. L. (2003). Mapping, modeling, and mentoring: Charting a course for professionalism in graduate medical education. *Cambridge Quarterly of Healthcare Ethics, 12*, 167–177.

Levy, B. T., Katz, J. T., Wolf, M. A., Sillman, J. S., Handen, R. I., & Dzau, V. J. (2004). An initiative in mentoring to promote residents' and faculty members' careers. *Academic Medicine, 79*(9), 845–850.

Lewis, R. J. (2003). Some thoughts regarding gender issues in the mentoring of future academicians. *Academic Emergency Medicine, 10*, 59–61.

Linzer, M., Visser, M. R. M., Oort, F. J., Smets, E. M. A., McMurray, J. E., & de Haes, H. C. J. M. (2001). Predicting and preventing physician burnout:

Results from the United States and the Netherlands. *American Journal of Medicine, 111,* 170–175.

Maheux, B., Beaudoin, C., Berkson, L., Cote, L., Des Marchais, J., & Jean, P. (2000). Medical faculty as humanistic physicians and teachers: The perceptions of students at innovative and traditional medical schools. *Medical Education, 34,* 630–634.

Maslach, C., & Jackson, S. E. (1986). *Maslach burnout inventory manual* (2nd ed.). Palo Alto, CA: Consulting Psychologists Press.

Masny, A., Ropka, M. E., Peterson, C., Fetzer, D., & Daly, M. B. (2008). Mentoring nurses in familial cancer risk assessment and counseling: Lessons learned from a formative evaluation. *Journal of Genetic Counseling, 17,* 196–207.

McNamara, B., Wadell, C., & Colvin, M. (1995). Threats to the good death: The cultural context of stress and coping among hospice nurses. *Sociology of Health and Illness, 17,* 222–244.

McPhaul, M. J. (2004). Issues in developing the medical scientist, part 2: Fostering research among medical students (interview with Michael John McPhaul, M.D.). *Journal of Investigative Medicine, 52,* 292–295.

Mintz, L. B., Bartels, K. M., & Rideout, C. A. (1995). Training in counseling ethnic minorities and race-based availability of graduate school resources. *Professional Psychology: Research and Practice, 26,* 316–321.

Mitchell, G. J. (2003). Nursing shortage or nursing famine: Looking beyond the numbers. *Nursing Science Quarterly, 16,* 219–224.

Morris, N., John, G., & Keen, T. (1988). Mentors learning the ropes. *Nursing Times, 84,* 24–27.

Myers Schim, S. (1990). Nursing career management: The Dalton/Thompson model. *Nursing Management, 21*(5), 97.

Nyquist, J. D. (2002). The PhD: A tapestry of change for the 21st century. *Change, 34*(6), 12–20.

Paglis, L. L., Green, S. G., & Bauer, T. N. (2006). Does adviser mentoring add value? A longitudinal study of mentoring and doctoral student outcomes. *Research in Higher Education, 47*(4), 451–476.

Papp, I., Markkanen, M., & von Bonsdorff, M. (2003). Clinical environment as a learning environment: Student nurses' perceptions concerning clinical learning experiences. *Nurse Education Today, 23,* 262–268.

Parkerson, G. R., Jr., Broadhead, W. E., & Tse, C. K. (1990). The health status and life satisfaction of first-year medical students. *Academic Medicine, 65,* 586–587.

Pascarella, E. T. (1980). Student-faculty informal contact and college outcomes. *Review of Educational Research, 50,* 545–595.

Pascarella, E. T., & Terezini, P. T. (1977). Patterns of student-faculty information interaction beyond the classroom and voluntary freshman attrition. *Journal of Higher Education, 48,* 540–552.

Perry, L. A. (1997). The Bridge Program: An overview. *Association of Black Nursing Faculty Journal, 8*(1), 4–7.

Petersdorf, R. G. (1986). The pathogenesis of fraud in medical science. *Annals of Internal Medicine, 104,* 252–254.

Phillips, R. M., Davies, W. B., & Neary, M. (1996a). The practitioner teacher: A study in the introduction of mentors in the preregistration nurse programme in Wales: Part 1. *Journal of Advanced Nursing, 23,* 1037–1044.

Phillips, R. M., Davies, W. B., & Neary, M. (1996b). The practitioner teacher: A study in the introduction of mentors in the preregistration nurse programme in Wales: Part 2. *Journal of Advanced Nursing, 23,* 1080–1088.

Pyskoty, C. E., Richman, J. A., & Flaherty, J. A (1990). Psychosocial assets and mental health of minority medical students. *Academic Medicine, 65,* 581–585.

Quaas, A. M., Berkowitz, L. R., & Tracy, E. E. (2009). Evaluation of a formal mentoring program in obstetrics and gynecology residency training program: Resident feedback and suggestions. *Journal of Graduate Medical Education, 1*(1), 132–138.

Ramanan, R. A., Taylor, W. C., Davis, R. B., & Phillips, R. S. (2006). Mentoring matters: Mentoring and career preparation in internal medicine residency training. *Journal of General Internal Medicine, 21,* 340–345.

Ramirez, A. J., Graham, J., Richards, M. A., Cull, A., & Gregory, W. M. (1996). Mental health of hospital consultants: The effects of stress and satisfaction at work. *Lancet, 347,* 724–728.

Rasmussen, B. H., Norberg, A., & Sandman, P. O. (1995). Stories about becoming a hospice nurse: Reasons, expectations, hopes and concerns. *Cancer Nursing, 18,* 344–354.

Rasmussen, B. H., Sandman, P. O., & Norberg, A. (1997). Stories about becoming a hospice nurse: A journey towards finding one's footing. *Cancer Nursing, 20,* 330–341.

Reynolds, P. F. (1994). Reaffirming professionalism through the education community. *Annals of Internal Medicine, 120,* 609–614.

Ricer, R. E., Fox, B. C., & Miller, K. E. (1995). Mentoring for medical students interested in family practice. *Family Medicine, 27,* 360–365.

Rogstad, K., & Talbot, M. (2001). A preliminary study comparing the attitudes of trainee doctors and their mentors to compulsory educational supervision in postgraduate medicine. *Mentoring & Tutoring, 9*(1), 77–83.

Rose, G. L., Rukstalis, M. R., & Schuckit, M. A. (2005). Informal mentoring between faculty and medical students. *Academic Medicine, 80*(4), 344–348.

Rosser, M., & King, L. (2003). Transition experiences of qualified nurses moving into hospice nursing. *Journal of Advanced Nursing, 43,* 206–215.

Shanafelt, T. D., Bradley, K. A., Wipf, J. E., & Back, A. L. (2002). Burnout and self-reported patient care in an internal medicine residency program. *Annals of Internal Medicine, 136,* 358–367.

Sirridge, M. S. (1985). The mentor system in medicine—How it works for women. *Journal of the American Medical Women's Association, 40*(2), 51–53.

Smith, P., & Gray, B. (2001). Reassessing the concept of emotional labour in student nurse education: The role of link lecturers and mentors in a time of change. *Nurse Education Today, 21,* 230–237.

Steiner, B. D., Pathman, D. E., Jones, B., Williams, E. S., & Riggins, T. (1999). Primary care physicians' training and their community involvement. *Family Medicine, 31*(4), 257–262.

Suen, L. K. P., & Chow, F. L. W. (2001). Students' perceptions of the effectiveness of mentors in an undergraduate nursing programme in Hong Kong. *Journal of Advanced Nursing, 36*(4), 505–511.

Taylor, R. B. (1980). The role of the academic adviser. *Journal of Medical Education, 55*, 216–217.

Tekian, A., Jalovecky, M. J., & Hruska, I. (2001). The impact of mentoring and advising at-risk underrepresented minority students on medical school performance. *Academic Medicine, 76*, 1264.

Tilghman, S. (1998). *Trends in the early careers of life scientists.* Report by the Committee on Dimensions, Causes and Implications of Recent Trends in the Careers of Life Scientists, National Research Council. Washington, DC: National Academy Press.

Tomanek, D., Moreno, N., Elgin, S. C., Flowers, S., May, V., Dolan, E., et al. (2005). Points of view: Effective partnerships between K-12 and higher education. *Cell Biology Education, 4*(1), 28–37.

Tracey, T. J., & Sedlacek, W. E. (1985). The relationship of noncognitive variables to academic success: A longitudinal comparison by race. *Journal of College Student Personnel, 26*, 405–410.

University of Michigan. (2006). *How to mentor graduate students: A guide for faculty at a diverse university.* MI: Regents of the University of Michigan.

University of Nebraska—Lincoln. (2009). *Graduate student mentoring guidebook.* Lincoln, NE: Author. Retrieved February 12, 2009, from http://www.unl.edu/gradstudies/current/dev/mentoring/common.shtml

University of Washington. (2005a). *Mentoring: How to mentor graduate students: A faculty guide.* Seattle, WA: The Graduate School, University of Washington.

University of Washington. (2005b). *Mentoring: How to mentor graduate students: A graduate student guide.* Seattle, WA: The Graduate School, University of Washington.

Waldeck, J. H., Orrego, V. O., Plax, T. G., & Kearney, P. (1997). Graduate student/faculty mentoring relationships: Who gets mentored, how it happens, and to what end. *Communication Quarterly, 45*(3), 93–109.

Weston, J. A., & Paterson, C. A. (1980). A medical school student support system at the University of Colorado School of Medicine. *Journal of Medical Education, 55*, 624–626.

Williams, B., & McLean, I. (1992). Someone to turn to. *Nursing Times, 18*(38), 48.

Wilson, R. C., Gaff, J. G., Dienst, E. R., Wood, L., & Bavry, J. L. (1975). *College professors and their impact on students.* New York: Wiley.

Wilson-Barnett, J., Butterworth, T., White, E., Twinn, S., Davies, S., & Riley, L. (1995). Clinical support and the project 2000 nursing student: Factors influencing this process. *Journal of Advanced Nursing, 21*, 1152–1158.

Woolnough, H. M., Davidson, M. J., & Fielden, S. L. (2006). The experiences of mentors on a career development and mentoring programme for female mental health nurses in the UK National Health Service. *Health Services Management Research, 19*, 186–196.

THREE

Case Study Three

Mentoring Roles With Students: Mental Health Training With a Community-Based Focus

Kathleen Clegg, Robert Ronis, and Martha Sajatovic

INTRODUCTION AND BACKGROUND

Over 80% of mental health expenditures dedicated to the treatment of individuals with mental health or substance abuse problems are *human resources*—the practitioners who provide and deliver mental health care (Blankertz & Robinson, 1997). It has been estimated that there were over half million clinically trained and active mental health professionals in the United States in 2002 (Manderscheid & Henderson, 2004). This work force includes a variety of disciplines including psychiatrists, psychologists, psychiatric social workers, counselors, and specialists in a variety of conditions such as substance abuse treatment and work in educational settings such as schools. However, currently more than half of mental health clinicians are over the age of 50, raising concerns regarding the adequacy of the current pipeline of trainees and young professionals to meet both the growing service demand and the approaching retirement of large segments of the workforce (Duffy et al., 2004).

Additional issues faced by the mental health professions are multiple and varied. Despite a good deal of attention to this issue over a number of years, there is still a substantial lack of cultural and racial diversity in the mental health workforce. The vast majority of mental health professionals are non-Hispanic Whites, who often exceed 90% of discipline composition (Duffy et al., 2004). Uneven geographic distribution of the mental health workforce, which is heavily concentrated in urban centers (Holzer, Goldsmith, & Ciarlo, 2000), offers another significant challenge. And there is a clear need for more mental health practitioners in community settings and neighborhoods where significant numbers of individuals with serious

99

mental disorders, such as schizophrenia and bipolar disorder, live and receive psychiatric care. Clearly, recruiting and training the next generation of mental health professionals must address these challenges, among others (Substance Abuse and Mental Health Services Administration, 2007).

Looking more closely at the discipline of psychiatry, in the United States today, the total number of psychiatrists is not increasing proportionately to the increase in the need for psychiatric services. The psychiatric workforce is aging with a mean age of 55 (Weissman, Sabshin, & Eist, 1999). Psychiatrists remain in particularly short supply in rural areas. Furthermore, in recent years, the number of minority medical graduates pursuing psychiatry training has been declining. Generally speaking, psychiatrists are spending less time with their patients due to increased patient volume expectations, predominance of medication management services, declining reimbursements, and greater paperwork burden. One bright spot is that women are pursuing the specialty in greater numbers.

Among those who have chosen psychiatry, many practice in community (public psychiatry) or managed care settings. The number of international medical graduates working in community/public sector psychiatry varies, but it is on the rise and is greater than 70% in some states (Weissman et al., 1999). Unfortunately, increasing numbers of psychiatrists who wish to offer psychotherapy as a treatment option have been finding it necessary to move away not just from public psychiatry, but also from taking insurance and other third party payments, relying instead on an almost exclusively "self pay" clientele.

A major concern regarding the preparation of the many needed future mental health professionals, including psychiatrists, is ensuring the availability and delivery of mentoring support and services to psychiatrists in training that can competently facilitate their professional development. This chapter will discuss mentoring medical students and residents, with a specific focus on the mentoring of psychiatrists in community settings and presentation of a successful, comprehensive model for training and mentoring that is being employed in the community.

OVERVIEW OF TRAINING FOR PSYCHIATRISTS

Although doctors have been taking care of persons with mental illness since the time of the ancient Greeks, psychiatry did not exist until the beginning of the 18th century (Shorter, 1997). Now with an accredited medical specialty, there are more than 120 psychiatry residency training programs in the United States alone (American Association of Directors of Psychiatric Residency Training, 2008). Because undergraduate medical education tends to be generic, offering only limited opportunities for medical students to pursue special interests during their fourth year, it is exclusively in these residency programs that the preparation of psychiatrists actually takes place.

The Accreditation Council for Graduate Medical Education (ACGME) lists specific requirements for psychiatry residency training: 4 years of postgraduate training, including 4 months of clinical rotations in internal medicine or another primary care area of practice; 2 months on neurology services; and training in inpatient and outpatient psychiatry. In the early years, most psychiatry residency programs, like the majority of medical training experiences at that time, employed an apprenticeship model. The term "resident" came into usage because the apprentices lived at the hospital to which they were assigned during this phase of their training.

As residency programs in psychiatry have since evolved, during the first year after graduation from medical school (the internship year), psychiatry residents are required to spend at least 4 months studying a primary care area, such as internal medicine, family medicine, or pediatrics; 2 months studying neurology; and the remaining 6 months studying psychiatry. Much of the time spent in psychiatry during the first year is spent working on inpatient psychiatric units in hospital settings, with attending psychiatrists as supervisors. Often, senior psychiatry residents provide additional supervision to interns. This model has trainees work with the sickest patients in the hospital setting during the earliest stage of their training; the model is not unique to psychiatry, but holds true for other medical specialties as well.

The second year of a psychiatry residency is often spent in the hospital setting, sometimes in specialty areas such as geropsychiatry (psychiatric practice with elderly patients), addiction psychiatry, or psychosomatic medicine. Second-year residents may also provide consultation-liaison services to medical and surgical patients in the hospital. In addition, second-year residents rotate through the emergency room, which provides them with an opportunity to practice evaluating in emergency setting patients who present with psychiatric symptoms.

It is not until the third year of psychiatry residency that residents begin to work with ambulatory patients. At this point, they have the opportunity to practice the psychotherapy skills they have been learning and to prescribe biologic and psychopharmacologic interventions for ambulatory patients. These ambulatory rotations can take place in a variety of settings, including hospital-based clinics, community mental health centers, Veterans Administration medical center clinics, university counseling centers, and/or private practice settings. During the third year of training, residents begin to have time to pursue elective areas of study that are of particular interest to them.

In the fourth and final year of their residencies, psychiatry residents have the option to pursue additional elective experiences that are consistent with their particular areas of interest. By the midpoint of the fourth year of residency, residents are also deeply involved in looking for employment following completion of the residency experience. Some choose to continue their training in a fellowship program in a psychiatric subspecialty, while others may pursue research, private practice, hospital-based practice, or the practice of public psychiatry in a community mental health center or state hospital setting.

Psychiatry Resident Background and Training Settings

American medical school graduates entering U.S. psychiatry residency programs come from both allopathic medical schools, granting the Doctor of Medicine (MD) degree, and osteopathic medical schools, granting the Doctor of Osteopathic Medicine (DO) degree. However, a rapidly growing proportion of those entering U.S. psychiatry residency programs are graduates of international medical schools. Psychiatry residencies located in larger urban areas on the east and west coasts tend to have higher percentages of U.S. medical graduates, while programs in smaller cities and more rural areas tend to have higher proportions of medical international graduates. The ratio of U.S. medical school graduates to international medical school graduates applying to and entering psychiatry residency programs varies greatly from one psychiatry residency to another.

Barriers to Pursuing Careers in Psychiatry

Many barriers exist to the pursuit of psychiatry as a career in medicine. As medical students graduate with increasing amounts of debt, smaller numbers of them are seeking the lower paid fields of medicine such as primary care and psychiatry. More students are pursuing specialties and subspecialties that include highly reimbursed "procedures" as an integral part of practice. On the other hand, many minority medical students may face pressure from family or community to pursue a medical specialty that is more "traditional" than psychiatry. International medical school graduates face an additional set of daunting challenges, including taking and passing the U.S. licensure examinations, obtaining a residency position, and passing the board certification examination, which international medical graduates have traditionally passed in lower numbers than graduates of U.S.-based medical schools.

THE MENTORING OF JUNIOR MEDICAL STUDENTS

Strong guidance and mentoring provided to "junior" medical students and recent graduates may help to mitigate and counteract some of the barriers to the selection of psychiatry as a career choice and as a choice for additional training, clinical practice, and/or research. Ideally, the mentorship of those potentially interested in psychiatry should begin early in their professional preparation, optimally during the first years of medical school.

As an example, medical students frequently begin to find mentors among the faculty who are involved in teaching courses during the first and second years of medical school, especially in courses that involve learning the clinical practice of medicine. Second year medical students potentially interested in psychiatry are exposed to a psychopathology curriculum and often seek out teachers who participate in delivering that curriculum as faculty mentors. At Case Western Reserve University School of Medicine, psychiatry residents are also involved in delivering the psychiatry curriculum and provide an additional pool of available mentors for such students.

During the third year of medical school, all students are required to have a psychiatry clerkship, which in the United States ranges from 3 to 8 weeks in length (Association of Directors of Medical Student Education in Psychiatry, 2008). During this clerkship experience, students have their first significant exposure to the practice of clinical psychiatry. It is here that trainees begin to see, learn about, and get a real "taste" of the practice of clinical psychiatry, and that their nascent interest in psychiatry may begin to emerge.

Many students do not become aware of their interest in psychiatry until they participate in a psychiatry clerkship. Relationships between students and faculty formed during the psychiatry clerkship experience can therefore be especially important in terms of the support and mentorship they offer to interested medical students. Psychiatry faculty members typically get to know such students quite well during the psychiatry clerkship and become a critical source of letters of recommendation when they later apply to psychiatry residency programs.

As indicated above, fourth year medical school students may pursue the specialties that most interest them and/or areas they feel will further prepare them to pursue their desired specialty training. During this time, some students do electives at hospitals affiliated with residency programs to which they are interested in applying, as a kind of "audition." This allows the student to learn more about the residency program and the residency program to evaluate the student. Students also prepare and submit their applications to residency programs during their fourth year of medical school, a process that can be very demanding. Consequently, it is very important that students have strong mentors who provide support, guidance, suggestions, and accurate feedback.

All students benefit during this period from strong coaching and/or mentoring by experienced, supportive faculty, who may assist trainees with the identification of their strengths, help them learn about the many career options available within the field of psychiatry, and offer support in dealing with self-imposed pressures, pressures from their families, and/ or pressures from their communities. Mentors with cultural backgrounds similar to those of their mentees may be particularly helpful, both with career choices and with the process.

THE MENTORING OF RESIDENTS

Mentorship Models for Psychiatry Trainees

There are a number of ways that faculty (full time, part-time, and adjunct) can mentor residents. These mentoring approaches can be classified into six broad categories or types of mentoring.

1. Support with Self-Assessment: This includes the identification of knowledge possessed, knowledge needed ("gaps"), skills, special strengths, weaknesses, blind spots, values, interests, preferences, learning style, cognitive style, and learning blocks.
2. Support for Career Search Activities: This includes the identification of possibilities (basic information about the many different careers that can be pursued within the field of psychiatry and its sub-specialties); identification and participation in reflective experiences; identification of questions and, ultimately, passions; and identification of other possible career-related mentors
3. Support with Mastering the Craft: This includes application and clarification of curricular content in basic science, communication, clinical reasoning, diagnosis, treatment, professionalism, ethics, practice-based learning, and improvement and systems-based practice.
4. Support with the Development of Cultural Competence: This includes expertise in interactions/relationships with patients and professional colleagues.
5. Emotional Support: This includes dealing with demanding placements, exams, application processes, feedback, and with particularly difficult or significantly altered personal circumstances and/or hardships.
6. Referral Source: This includes the identification of learning resources and learning resource persons for all of the above, and the cultivation of initiative and resourcefulness in trainees in their pursuit of such resources.

With residents, most mentoring is accomplished during and by way of supervision and coaching interactions. This breadth and depth of the mentor–mentee relationship requires that the mentor address multiple objectives simultaneously in an integrated manner. Some examples of this sort of fusion of multiple objectives and agendas will be illustrated in the vignettes described further on in this chapter. While the vignettes presented address cultural issues faced by residents coming from cultural contexts that differed from those of their colleagues and/or patients, it can be seen that multiple objectives and issues were present, and multiple types of mentoring were needed to be provided by the mentor, in each situation.

Notwithstanding the need to fuse multiple types of mentoring, it is worth noting that in the current climate in which mentors face numerous simultaneous demands on their time and mentees require various dimensions of support, trainees are constantly finding and adding mentors. Trainees no longer need to think of themselves as depending on a single person as their mentor. Therefore, any one mentor is relieved of the pressure to try to "do it all." Rather, the mentor in this and in any similar contexts should strive to be mindful of his/her own limitations and the importance of referring students to other resource persons and mentors when and as needed.

Socialization to the Profession of Psychiatry and Development of Cultural Competence: The Public Academic Liaison (PAL) Program, a Model Program Facilitating Comprehensive Socialization to the Practice of Community Psychiatry

The PAL Program features an innovative collaboration between the Department of Psychiatry at University Hospitals Case Medical Center/ Case Western Reserve University School of Medicine and the Cuyahoga County Community Mental Health Board. Cuyahoga County's Board is one of 53 local mental health services boards responsible for local planning and resource allocation under Ohio's decentralized community mental health system. Based in Cleveland, Ohio, and established in 1990, PAL was created with two primary missions in mind: (1) to provide an organized, faculty-supervised experience in interdisciplinary community mental health services for trainees in residency training at University Hospitals, and (2) to provide needed high-quality psychiatric services and a conduit for the recruitment of future psychiatry graduates into the local service system (Brauzer, Lefley, & Steinbook, 1996; Blankertz & Robinson (1997); Goetz et al., 1998; Ronis, 1992; Santos et al., 1994; Svendsen et al., 2005; Tucker, 1995).

Third and fourth year residents are assigned to one of several designated training sites among the 37 agencies supported by the Board, and spend 1 day each week over the course of 1 or 2 years providing services at their assigned sites. A faculty supervisor is assigned to work side-by-side with each resident. Faculty members also provide direct patient services in addition to the individual case supervision they provide to residents. Faculty members organize and conduct a supervision/teaching session at the end of each such day. Initially, all supervisors were full-time faculty members from the University who accompanied the residents to their site locations. More recently, (volunteer) clinical faculty, who are most often graduates of the PAL program who have been retained as Medical Directors or full-time clinicians by the agencies, have been added to the ranks and have increased the availability of on-site PAL supervisors.

Clinical services provided by the residents are similar to those they perform in their outpatient clinics at the University, including psychiatric assessments and medication management follow-up visits. Occasionally, residents may participate in groups or provide individual psychotherapy to selected patients at these community sites, but the emphasis is on the specialized services that a community psychiatrist provides within the context of a multidisciplinary team of case managers, social workers, psychologists, and others. Most patients served by PAL suffer from serious mental illnesses (SMI) associated with long-term disability, such as schizophrenia, schizoaffective disorders, bipolar disorders, and major depression. Many also have co-occurring substance use disorders and/or physical illnesses as a focus of their treatment. Comorbidity is the norm.

In their PAL placements, residents participate in multidisciplinary team meetings and case conferences, and collaborate with nonphysician team members in their assessments and management of these seriously ill and often medically indigent patients. They become familiar with the range and limitations of community resources and with the operations of the service systems ranging from state hospital to rehabilitation and housing, and become attuned to the social and cultural characteristics of their patients. Occasional home visits by the resident physician are encouraged. However, in practice, the pressing need for doctor time at agencies usually severely limits or precludes resident time being devoted to this purpose.

An ongoing series of community case conferences is held in order to bring trainees and a variety of mentors together, on a monthly basis, in order to discuss clinical cases from various settings in the community and from diverse professional perspectives. In these community case conferences, residents have the opportunity to see patients with varied psychiatric diagnoses and backgrounds and to interact with different faculty mentors. Staff at the agencies also benefit from the opportunity to receive on-site education from visiting faculty, alongside the psychiatry residents and to participate actively in case discussions.

Supplemental clinical activities are provided through participation in a "Community Block" rotation; over the years, this has included services at a 2-week residential treatment Crisis Stabilization Program, with the Adult Mobile Crisis Team, the county Psychiatric Emergency Services program, and a number of other community settings. The additional elective offerings that are available are frequently sought after by advanced residents and provide further opportunity for career search experiences, beyond that provided by the primary PAL placement.

Since its inception, the PAL program has grown to include Child and Adolescent Psychiatry trainees and fellows in our Geriatric, Forensic, and Addiction programs. A Community Psychiatry Fellowship was established in 1998, which is comprised of 30 hours of clinical services and supplemental clinical and administrative teaching opportunities. Since 1990 more than 150 general and child psychiatry residents have participated in the PAL program, and together with faculty supervisors have provided more than 200,000 hours of direct clinical services through the agencies of the Cuyahoga County system.

While the Public Academic Liaison (PAL) program model provides close on-site supervision by a PAL faculty member for all resident trainees, this support is particularly important in the case of internationally trained mental health trainees. Differences in cultural background from the client population, as well as the community mental health center staff, can be particularly challenging for international medical graduates.

In addition to the on-site supervision in community mental health centers settings, the residents also receive formal didactic sessions relevant to community mental health topics. These include working as part of an interdisciplinary team, working with homeless individuals, working with individuals presenting in crisis, and working with clients with co-morbid substance use disorders and psychiatric illness. All residents participate in didactic sessions and workshops on cultural psychiatry topics, which explore the complexity of interactions between mental health providers and clients of different cultural backgrounds, a challenge for all psychiatry residents, and again particularly so for residents who are international medical graduates.

Socialization to the Profession on an Individual Basis

While the following case vignette examples focus on community psychiatry resident trainees, the mentorship concepts could apply to mentorship of other mental health trainees as well. The multiple types of mentoring addressed in each vignette are identified; however, these case examples all illustrate and focus on the challenges related to cultural differences between mental health providers and their patients and the opportunities to support the development of cultural competence in residents that they present.

THE CASE OF DR. A. Dr. A, a 26-year-old Asian psychiatry graduate of medical school in his native country, found it particularly challenging to participate in the interdisciplinary team model that is utilized in U.S. community mental health centers. His personal cultural background, as well as medical training, was more consistent with the role of the medical doctor as the leader of the team and the ultimate authority on all matters related to the care of the patient. Dr. A's preference was to see clients alone, not allowing case managers to sit in on the patient's appointment. He became defensive when team members gave him information about the patient, feeling as though his primary role in the care of the patient was being questioned.

Through mentoring that supported self-assessment, Dr. A's mastery of key aspects of the craft, and the development of cultural competence, Dr. A began to see the value of the interdisciplinary team, particularly when information critical to the care of the client was made available, such as information about the client's drug and alcohol use. Mentoring this resident involved helping him to understand both the impact of his own cultural background and the different model pursued in the United States, a model that is not inherently better or worse than that with which he was accustomed, but different. This understanding allowed him to maintain his personal integrity and pride in his cultural background, while making the adaptations necessary to function as a part of an interdisciplinary team.

THE CASE OF DR. B. Dr. B was a 27-year-old female physician of Russian background, who had graduated from medical school in her native country. Initially, Dr. B found it difficult to function effectively as a member of an interdisciplinary care team. Dr. B also became frustrated with clients who were nonadherent with their treatment plans. She felt she could not be helpful to the client if he/she did not follow her advice and prescriptions.

Mentoring required taking a particularly egalitarian, collaborative approach with this resident, and avoiding as far as possible the "expert/ student" model, which would have been counterproductive. Through mentoring that supported self-assessment, mastery of the craft, and the development of cross-cultural competence and emotional support, the resident was helped to identify factors that influenced her ability to function in a community mental health center. These included resistance on her part to rules or policies that made her feel that she was being "told what to do." Over time, she learned how to function in a more collaborative way with other members of the community mental health center interdisciplinary team. She began to develop more effective relationships with clients, including those who at times were not adherent to prescribed medications or other aspects of the treatment plan. She was able to more fully appreciate the dynamics of being "told what to do" that clients may experience. She gradually learned to develop a treatment plan in collaboration with the client, after eliciting the client's goals and priorities.

THE CASE OF DR. C. Dr. C was a 30-year-old man of Middle Eastern background who attended medical school in his native country. He admitted that due to his cultural and religious background, further reinforced by his medical training, he viewed drug and alcohol abuse as a moral weakness. He found it difficult to embrace the disease model of drug and alcohol abuse that is widely ascribed to and utilized in the United States. When a client relapsed on drugs or alcohol, Dr. C initially felt that treatment with him should be terminated, as the client had violated the treatment contract.

Through mentoring that supported self-assessment, mastery of addiction medicine content, and development of cultural competence, and provided emotional support, Dr. C was able to acknowledge that his attitudes toward such clients were due to his sense of helplessness and his own anger at clients for relapsing, which he previously had seen as a weakness on the client's part. Education regarding the disease model had not initially been sufficient to "widen his lens." In the context of a trusting, respectful mentorship relationship, however, he was able to recognize and acknowledge his own cultural and religious beliefs. While these values guided his personal choices and behaviors, he learned to separate these from his role as a mental health professional. The successful mentoring relationship had to be nonjudgmental, in order to help the resident to become less judgmental. This newfound perspective allowed Dr. C to collaborate with his clients on a plan of care that addressed issues that were of importance to the clients.

THE CASE OF DR. D. Dr. D, an American medical graduate from a U.S. medical school, began residency training in internal medicine and transferred into a psychiatry residency after her internship year. Dr. D found it difficult to make the shift from a specialty where diagnoses can be more easily and frequently confirmed through laboratory and clinical findings to the relative ambiguity of psychiatric diagnoses. She was surprised and dismayed by psychiatry's negative stigma within the medical community as a whole.

Through mentoring that supported self-assessment, provided emotional support, and modeled successful strategies adopted by her mentor, Dr. D was able to learn methods of coping with this stigma. She was able to see that the stigma against psychiatry as a profession reflects the stigma that exists against mental illness in general and psychiatric patients specifically. United States-born residents also face cultural differences and cultural competence issues in the care of their psychiatry patients, often due to differences in ethnic background or differing socioeconomic status. It may be difficult for the resident, who may have grown up in a privileged home, as was the case for this resident, to understand the difficulties faced by patients living in poverty. A successful mentoring relationship that supported the resident's self-assessment and development of cultural competence (in this case, understanding the lived context of those who are in poverty) helped this resident examine her tacit assumptions and beliefs, as well as the limited range of possibilities most public psychiatry patients face.

There are numerous similar examples of the impact of PAL mentor on the development of cultural and other competencies in the residents they supervise. The PAL program model of on-site one-on-one supervision of residents, periodic case conferences, and complementary didactics, is particularly suited to addressing the conflicts that arise in "real time," whether due to differences in culture, personal preferences and style, professional judgment, or a host of other factors. It is in the actual clinical situation that trainees are most open to learning, making it an ideal setting for mentorship and supervision.

An Additional Note on PAL Career Search Mentoring

Many psychiatry residents participating in the PAL program identify specific interests, possibly subspecialty interests, over the course of their training. Some residents have developed further interest in community psychiatry and a subset of these also have an interest in the administrative aspects of public psychiatry systems of care. Others develop interest in subspecialty areas such as forensic psychiatry, addiction psychiatry, emergency psychiatry, or women's mental health. Awareness of these developing interests by the faculty supervisor/mentor allows the mentor to help shape the resident's caseload of patients to include clients that present with these issues.

PAL supervisors routinely invite the residents they supervise to discuss their future career plans and, when appropriate, possible future steps they might want to take in the way of additional training, such as a fellowship. Obviously, when a resident's interests differ from the interests and/or expertise of the mentor, the mentor needs to possess the self-awareness, self-confidence, and integrity to support the resident in pursuing his or her area(s) of interest without undue influence toward a particular area of study, and more affirmatively, to direct the resident to other possible mentors in the area(s) of the resident's own choosing.

MENTORSHIP IN RESEARCH AND SCHOLARLY ACTIVITIES WITH A COMMUNITY-BASED FOCUS

In 2001, The National Institute of Mental Health (NIMH) established a bibliography of brain and behavioral research studies for a national mental health conference (NIMH, 2001). A review of a randomly selected subset of 249 papers from this bibliography indicates that one-half of the first authors were psychiatrists. A further review of the same subset of papers was conducted by independent lay reviewers. Sixty percent of the papers identified by these lay reviewers as most important to the future of public mental health listed psychiatrists as first authors. This informal assessment demonstrated that psychiatrists have a substantive presence on projects and publications that are considered valuable to the national research agenda and the broader public as well. Unfortunately, in spite of the rapid and important growth in behavioral health research in the past decade, there is an identified shortage of psychiatrist researchers in the United States that begins with a limited number of trainees who develop research interest and expertise and extends into a shortage of trained psychiatrist researchers (Research Training in Psychiatry Residency, 2003). Only 15% of faculty at U.S. medical schools spend more than one-half of their time in research and fewer than 2% of all U.S. psychiatrists have research as their primary activity (Abrams, Patchan, & Boat, 2003; American Association of Medical Colleges, 2002). Clearly, additional researchers are needed to move the field forward in developing, testing, and evaluating mental health treatments and technology.

It has been suggested that increasing the number of research trainees and subsequent numbers of psychiatrist-trained personnel in the mental health research workforce hinges upon enhancing research opportunities and interest during psychiatric training (Abrams et al., 2003). Because psychiatric residency programs vary in terms of size, focus, and local expertise, programs might deliver a range of basic research literacy that begins with basic research/scholarly skills (expertise with interpreting the scientific literature, understanding the basis of evidence-based practice) and extends to more sophisticated programming that trains large numbers of patient-oriented psychiatrist researchers such as institutions that provide advanced fellowship training in research methodologies (Abrams et al., 2003).

The National Institute of Mental Health (NIMH) has explained how psychiatry residency programs might improve their residency-based research training. Recommendations include (1) hiring of faculty and staff who are explicitly dedicated to research mentoring and training, (2) acquiring and providing equipment and facilities for research training, (3) facilitating the implementation of short-term or pilot research activities and projects by trainees, and (4) including research training across the full range of psychiatry training including adult and child/adolescent residency and fellowship training. All of these measures can be applied in the service of enhancing and improving public or community mental health research. Additionally, training programs that have a strong clinical community psychiatry presence, such as the PAL program, and appropriate mentoring support for psychiatry research are likely to attract trainees who can be developed into future community mental health researchers.

It is to be expected that research training for residents and fellows in psychiatry must deal with many of the same issues that have been previously discussed in socialization to the profession of psychiatry: cultural mismatch between trainees and clinical research populations, development of the ability to work in multidisciplinary teams, and solidification of professional identity. In addition, research is often an endeavor that is not compensated with financial or professional success early on in one's career. Appropriate mentoring and support can be helpful in providing nonsalary benefits for trainees, such as a supportive network of colleagues and supervisors and facilitated opportunities to participate in scientific advances. Additional promotion strategies to increase the number of community mental health researchers might include financial incentives such as loan repayment programs to those trainees who commit to research involvement beyond minimal clinical training requirements. However, this type of approach would clearly require collaboration between training programs, which are typically clinically based, and those entities invested in strengthening the pipeline of young investigators, such as NIMH.

Finally, professional organizations such as the American Psychiatry Association (APA) provide additional opportunities for training and mentoring in research. The American Psychiatric Institute for Research and Education (APIRE) provides a number of research training opportunities, including a research colloquium for junior investigators that heavily features research mentorship, the facilitation of links to research fellowships among leading academic departments of psychiatry, and the granting of research training awards and research awards (American Psychiatry Association, 2009). Both the APA and NIMH have programs that emphasize the training of minorities, women, and investigators that have traditionally been underrepresented in the research workforce, and may present opportunities to train and promote the development of investigators in public or community mental health as well.

CONCLUSION

Mentoring plays a key role in training mental health clinicians and researchers with a community-based or public health focus. While the challenges are many, including resource barriers and a relative scarcity of comprehensive models for training and mentoring that can be employed in the community, the rewards and benefits of successful mentoring are high. Ultimately, successful mentoring will produce an increase in the number of skilled clinicians and researchers in the field of community mental health.

REFERENCES

Abrams, M. T., Patchan, K., & Boat, T. F. (Eds.). (2003). *Research training in psychiatry residency: Strategies for Reform Committee on Incorporating Research into Psychiatry Residency*. Washington, DC: The National Academies Press.

American Association of Directors of Psychiatric Residency Training. (2008). Retrieved March 12, 2009, from http://www.aadprt.org/

American Association of Medical Colleges. (2002). *AAMC data book: Statistical information related to medical education*. Washington, DC: Association of Medical Colleges.

American Psychiatry Association. (2009). Retrieved March 12, 2009, from http://www.psych.org

Association of Directors of Medical Student Education in Psychiatry. (2008). Retrieved March 12, 2009, from http://www.admsep.org/

Blankertz, L. E., & Robinson, S. E. (1997). Recruitment and retention of psychosocial rehabilitation workers. *Administration & Policy in Mental Health, 24*(3), 221–234.

Brauzer, B., Lefley H. P., & Steinbook, R. (1996). A module for training residents in public mental health systems and community resources. *Psychiatric Services, 47*(2), 192–194.

Duffy, F. F., West, J. C., Wilk, J., Narrow, W. E., Hales, D., Thompson, J., et al. (2004). Mental health practitioners and trainees. In R. W. Manderscheid & M. J. Henderson (Eds.), *Mental health, United States, 2002* (pp. 327–368) [DHHS Publication No. SMA 04-3938]. Rockville, MD: U.S. Department of Health and Human Services, Substance Abuse and Mental Health Services Administration, Center for Mental Health Services.

Goetz, R., Cutler, D. L., Pollack, D., Falk, N., Birecree, E., McFarland, et al. (1998). A three-decade perspective on community and public psychiatry training in Oregon. *Psychiatric Services, 49*(9), 1208–1211.

Holzer, C. E., III., Goldsmith, H. F., & Ciarlo, J. A. (2000). The availability of health and mental health providers by population density. *Journal of the Washington Academy of Sciences, 86*(3), 25–33.

Manderscheid, R. W., & Henderson, M. J. (Eds.). (2004). *Mental health, United States, 2002* (DHHS Publication No. SMA-04-3938). Rockville, MD: U.S. Department of Health and Human Services, Substance Abuse and Mental Health Services Administration, Center for Mental Health Services.

National Institute of Mental Health. (2001). *Science on our minds*. Retrieved March 12, 2009, from http://www.nimh.nih.gov

Ronis, R. (1992). Public Academic Liaison (PAL): Community service and education through creative collaboration. *Innovations and Research, 1*, 3.

Substance Abuse and Mental Health Services Administration. (2007). *An action plan for behavioral workforce development—a framework for discussion*. Retrieved January 16, 2009, from www.samhsa.gov/workforce/annapolis/workforceactionplan.pdf

Santos, A. B., Ballenger, J. C., Bevilacqua, J. J., Zealberg, J. J., Hiers, T. G., McLeod-Bryant, S., et al. (1994). A community-based public-academic liaison program. *American Journal of Psychiatry, 151*(8), 1181–1187.

Shorter, E. (1997). *A history of psychiatry: From the era of the asylum to the age of Prozac.* New York: John Wiley & Sons.

Svendsen, D., Cutler, D. L., Ronis, R. J., Herman, L. C, Morrison, A., Smith M, et al. (2005). The professor of public psychiatry model in Ohio: The impact on training, program innovation and quality of mental health care. *Community Mental Health Journal, 41*(6), 775–784.

Tucker, W. (1995). Public-academic liaisons in psychiatric residency training in New York State. *Psychiatric Services, 46*(12), 1289–1291.

Weissman, S. H., Sabshin, M., & Eist, H. (1999). *Psychiatry in the new millenium.* Washington, DC: American Psychiatric Publishing.

FOUR

Diversity Issues
in the Context of Mentoring

DEFINING DIVERSITY

Diversity has been defined as

> attitudes, beliefs, and hence, behaviors, of individuals [which] are socially
> constructed within a context of group and intergroup relations and ... people
> act through social, political, and economic institutions that create, embed,
> and reproduce the inequality among people which we then call diversity.
> Diversity is then acted out in the practices of everyday life and interpreted
> through lenses of moral and ethical reasoning that, when unexamined, legit-
> imate both unearned privilege and unearned disadvantage. The origin of
> diversity, however, is not in the reactions to differences in daily interaction ...
> but rather diversity is created and perpetuated in the historical, institutional,
> cultural, and hence, moral, construction of difference and is reinforced by the
> structures of opportunity, resources, and power. While there may be "real"
> differences rooted in biology, we would argue that the dimensions of such
> differences are unknowable, given the filtering and conditioning that occurs
> through interaction with culture, history, and social institutions. (DiTomaso &
> Hooijberg, 1996, pp. 164–165)

This definition recognizes that the concept of diversity and issues
associated with diversity arise not only from superficial differences,
such as skin color, but from the interactions between those who perceive
difference and those who are perceived to embody such differences.
Accordingly, the concept of diversity can be construed broadly to include
race, ethnicity, sex, gender, sexual orientation, religion, and national origin
or citizenship.

Issues relating to diversity in the context of mentoring health
professionals are important for several reasons. As of 2002, minorities
constituted 27% of the U.S. population (Hobbs & Stoops, 2002). It is estimated that by the year 2050, persons of color will constitute 48% of the
national population. Despite these population changes, U.S. minorities
continue to be underrepresented in higher education programs in the
sciences and health professions. Racial and ethnic minorities receive
only 16% of the undergraduate degrees and 9% of the doctoral degrees
in science and engineering (Crowley, Fuller, Law, McKeon, & Ramirez,

2004; Olson & Fagan, 2007). Although there are approximately 2.9 million licensed registered nurses in the United States, only 10.7% claim minority status (United States Department of Health and Human Services, Health Resources and Services Administration, 2006). Of these, only 4.9% are African American, 3.7% are Asian or Pacific Islander, 0.5% are American Indian or Alaskan Native, and only 2.0% are Latino. In 2006, only 7.3% of the membership of the American Speech-Language-Hearing Association, consisting of speech and language pathologists, audiologists, and speech, language, and hearing scientists, reported minority status (Wright-Harp & Cole, 2008). By 2009, the proportion had decreased to 6.9%, compared to 24.9% of the U.S. population (American Speech-Language-Hearing Association, 2010). A reported decrease in the number of minority applicants entering medical school has also raised concerns (Hayes, 2006). In particular, the number of minority men entering graduate and professional schools and receiving doctoral and professional degrees has failed to increase significantly (American Council of Education, 2006). Minorities are similarly underrepresented among researchers receiving funding from the National Institutes of Health (Walters & Simoni, 2009; Wyatt, Williams, Henderson, & Sumner, 2009).

Disparity in the numbers of women and men entering specific health professions is also of concern. Although the numbers of women receiving advanced degrees in science and medicine have increased over the years (Malcolm, Chubin, & Jesse, 2004; Salsberg & Grover, 2006), girls and women continue to be discouraged from entering the fields of science, technology, engineering, and mathematics (STEM) (Committee on the Guide to Recruiting and Advancing Women Scientists and Engineers in Academia, National Research Council, 2006). In some health professions, such as speech pathology and other areas of human communication sciences and disorders, there has been a steady decline of male professionals (Tonkovich & Slater, 2004). As of 2009, males represented only 4.2% of speech-language pathologists, 18.2% of audiologists, and 26.6% of individuals with dual certification (American Speech-Language-Hearing Association, 2010).

This underrepresentation of racial and ethnic minorities in the health professions and the lack of proportionate gender representation in some of the health professions have been attributed, in part, to a lack of mentoring (Nettles & Millett, 2006). Results from a nationwide survey of doctoral programs found that although 70% of all doctoral students had a mentor, more than one-third of African Americans in science and mathematics did not have a mentor (Nettles & Millett, 2002). Study findings have indicated that faculties were often reluctant to mentor racial/ethnic minority students because of their lower GRE scores, lower undergraduate grade point averages, and graduation from less prestigious universities (Nettles & Millett, 2002).

The difficulties encountered by U.S. racial and ethnic minorities and women may be compounded for students and health professions arriving to the United States from other countries. An increasing proportion of health care professionals who are training and/or practicing in the United States, often on a temporary basis, have been educated outside this country. Many may be members of U.S-identified minority groups and/or may be unfamiliar with U.S. culture or the values that underlie the U.S. health care system. As an example, for some years the United States has experienced a critical shortage of trained nurses (American Association of Colleges of Nursing, 2010). This shortage has been eased periodically through the establishment of federal immigration procedures designed to facilitate the temporary immigration of nurses from the Philippines and other countries to the United States (Herbst, 2009). Similarly, U.S. immigration law displays greater leniency toward those foreign medical graduates wishing to practice in the United States who commit to doing so in medically underserved areas for specified periods of time (Dovlo, 2005).

The increased availability of effective mentoring for students and faculty from minority groups at all stages of education, beginning with secondary school and extending through college and professional training, could yield numerous benefits not only to the mentees themselves, but also to our larger society: a broadening of the research agenda; an increase in our knowledge of particular communities, which is necessary to address existing health problems; and an increase in the availability and provision of culturally competent care (Stoff, Forsyth, Marquez, & McClure, 2009; Treadwell, Braithwaite, Braithwaite, Oliver, & Holliday, 2009; Walters & Simoni, 2009). The relative scarcity of culturally competent care now available is adversely impacting minority individuals and their larger communities. Research continues to suggest that existing health disparities between majority and underrepresented minority populations that are educationally and economically comparable are attributable, at least in part, to continuing racial or ethnic prejudice on the part of providers (Bach, 2003; Ford, 2004; Smedley, Stith, & Nelson, 2003).

RACE, ETHNICITY, AND MENTORING

Race, Ethnicity, and Mentoring Students

Research indicates that many students from underrepresented minority (URM) groups, including African Americans, Latinos, Asians and Pacific Islanders, and American Indians/Alaskan Natives forego attending graduate school due to disillusionment and unpleasant experiences during the course of their secondary and undergraduate schooling (Lang, 1986). For example, African American students at predominantly White institutions may often face issues of socialization, isolation, and marginalization (D'Augelli & Hershberger, 1993; Fries-Britt & Turner, 2002). These issues, which arise directly from the students' underrepresentation, have been identified as obstacles to the professional success of African American male medical students (Odom, Roberts, Johnson, & Cooper, 2007). First-generation college students are at especially high risk of attrition from higher education (Terrell & Hassell, 1994). These different experiences may be attributable to the different historical and structural positions they hold both inside and outside of the educational institution, to a lack of familiarity with the university environment, and to the absence of a family tradition of higher education (Cropper, 2000). Existing stereotypes about minority students and their lack of aspiration and their disinterest in higher education may erect barriers in accessing faculty members and fellow students, thereby interfering with the minority students' ability to succeed (Rivera-Goba & Nieto, 2007). (Stereotypes are addressed in additional detail further in this chapter.) Additional challenges to the pursuit of higher education toward both clinical and research careers in health include a lack of financial aid, a lack of adequate preparation for higher education, the need for health benefits and family support that take precedence over continued training, and a lack of emotional support from within the academic institution (Campbell & Davis, 1996; Grumbach, Coffman, Rosenoff, & Muñoz, 2001; Sedlacek, 1999; Villaruel, Canales, & Torres, 2001; Wyatt et al., 2009).

It has been suggested that the difficulties encountered by minority students can be somewhat ameliorated through the development of a mentoring relationship with a mentor of the same race. Mentors and mentees who share key characteristics may feel a shared sense of identity and have a higher level of comfort with each other (Ragins, 1997), dynamics that may positively affect the quality of and extent to which the mentor provides the mentee with assistance related to career development and psychosocial support; this, in turn, may positively influence the career outcomes of the mentee, such as promotion, career aspirations, and career satisfaction (Ragins, 1997).

However, there are relatively few minority faculties at institutions of higher learning (Rivera-Goba & Nieto, 2007). As an example, African Americans constitute just 5.3% of all full-time faculties at American colleges and universities, although they represent 60% of all faculties at historically Black colleges and universities (*Journal of Blacks in Higher Education*, 2007). In the college and university setting, Latino faculty holding doctoral degrees constituted only 1.9% of the members of the American Speech-Language Hearing Association who reported a non-White racial/ethnic background (Wright-Harp & Cole, 2008).

It is possible that heterogeneity in key characteristics, such as ethnicity or sex, between the mentor and the mentee may reflect power imbalances within the larger organization and/or society and may be associated with differing degrees of mentoring functions. Nevertheless, research has produced inconsistent findings with respect to the effectiveness of same-race mentoring as compared with cross-race or cross-cultural mentoring inconsistent. Studies have found a positive correlation between the presence of minority teachers in secondary schools and the number of minority students who matriculated into college (Hess & Leal, 1997). Meznek, McGrath, and Galaviz (1989) suggested that same-race mentors are able to address more effectively conflicts that may exist between the values of a student's culture or community and those of the educational institution. Consistent with other researchers (Thomas, 1990), Koberg, Bosos, and Goodman (1998) reported from their study with 367 men and women employed in diverse health professions that protégés received greater levels of psychosocial mentoring from mentors of the same race compared with those who have mentors of a different race. Mentors of the same race or ethnicity can serve as role models (Rivera-Goba & Nieto, 2007) and exemplify one's ability to succeed in higher education while still maintaining a positive sense of one's racial or ethnic identity, in essence, to be both equal and different (Cropper, 2000). Frierson, Hargrove, and Lewis (1994) found that Black students paired with Black mentors reported more positive interactions with their mentors than did Black students who had been paired with White mentors.

However, attempts to match mentors and mentees on the basis of perceived similarities are not unproblematic. In many mentoring programs, a third party is responsible for matching the mentor with an appropriate mentee; this is often done on the basis of perceived shared characteristics, in the belief that these similarities will facilitate the development of a successful mentoring experience. The process of matching must be recognized as an enactment of power with potentially significant implications:

> The effective categorization of a group of people by a more powerful "other" is not therefore "just" a matter of classification (if, indeed, there is such a thing). It is necessarily an intervention in that group's social world which will, to an extent and in ways that are a function of the specifics of the situation, alter that world and the experience of living in it. . . . [A] concern with external definition and categorization demands that we pay attention to *power* and *authority*, and the manner in which different modes of domination are implicated in the social construction of ethnic and other identities . . . . (Jenkins, 2003, p. 69)

Accordingly, how individuals self-identify may vary depending upon the social, historical, and political context in which the designation is to be made (Tajfel & Turner, 1986); their self-designation may vary during the course of their lives, as one or more of subidentities, such as sex, gender, religion, ethnicity, race, or culture, becomes increasingly salient.

Consequently, the characteristic(s) utilized for matching the mentors and the mentees by a third party may not mirror the characteristic that the individuals themselves use as the basis of their self-identity.

Further, research teams have also reported that African American students place greater importance on the quality of the mentoring relationship than the race of their mentor (Lee, 1999; Wallace, Abel, & Ropers-Huilman, 2000). A study involving African American and non-Hispanic White social workers found that although mentors and mentees tended to select each other on the basis of race, there was no indication that perceptions of the quality of the mentoring relationship differed on the basis of racial concordance (Collins, Kamya, & Tourse, 2001). Researchers reported from their retrospective survey of minority members of the American Psychological Association that ethnic similarities between mentors and their mentees were unrelated to mentees' ratings of perceived benefits (Atkinson, Neville, & Casas, 1991). A survey study involving 170 mostly African American graduates of Howard University's School of Business, including individuals working in medicine and health services, found that those individuals who had established mentoring relationships with White male mentors experienced compensation advantages compared to those graduates who had never formed mentoring relationships and those whose mentors were not White males (Dreher & Chargois, 1998).

These findings do not suggest that minority students should seek out only minority mentors if they wish to experience an effective mentoring relationship or that the students should seek developmental relationships only with White male mentors if they wish to advance in their careers. Rather, these data suggest that the effectiveness of the mentoring relationship and the participants' satisfaction with the relationship likely rest on how issues of racial/ethnic differences are addressed within the mentoring relationship.

Although both the mentor and the mentee bear responsibility to address these issues (Davidson & Foster-Johnson, 2001), this exchange is not merely a discussion between two individuals. Rather,

> what should be a simple matter of negotiation between two persons becomes an arbitration between historical legacies, contemporary racial tensions, and societal protocols. A cross-cultural mentoring relationship is an affiliation between unequals who are conducting their relationship on a hostile American stage, with a societal script contrived to undermine the success of the partnership. (Johnson-Bailey & Cervero, 2002, p. 18)

The success of and satisfaction with the mentoring relationship ultimately depends on openness in the discussion of these issues (Johnson-Bailey & Cervero, 2002; Thomas, 1993); the development of trust on an individual level; and a recognition and acknowledgement that the mentor and the mentee may experience their institutional environment in vastly different ways due to differences in race, ethnicity, and life experience (Johnson-Bailey & Cervero, 2002).

A variety of mentoring models can be utilized in addition to or instead of the classic model of mentoring. Cropper (2000) has suggested that a carefully matched peer mentor, rather than a faculty mentor, can provide a student with personal support, can help to raise consciousness, can take a proactive role in the student's development as a minority professional, and can assist the mentee in developing a network. Unlike a faculty–student mentoring relationship, a peer mentoring relationship also permits a greater sharing of power between the mentor and the mentee. The peer mentors can be supported through regular meetings and the development of a system to facilitate feedback to management. This model has been found to be beneficial to both the mentees and the peer mentors in a social work program.

Rabionet, Santiago, and Zorrilla (2009) have suggested the use of a multifaceted mentoring model of minority health researchers that includes the establishment of multi-institutional collaborations, the creation of a systematic training program based on competency development in identified core areas, and the creation and nurturing of cross-disciplinary teams that include both the mentors and the mentees. Continuing periodic activities, such as retreats, conferences, meetings, and workshops help to ensure the sustainability of the professional and personal relationships that are developed through this mentoring process.

As noted in Chapter 1, the Peer-Onsite-Distance approach to multi-level mentoring has been found to be effective as a mentoring strategy with underrepresented minority medical school faculty (Lewellen-Williams et al., 2006). Mentors include peers, who provide collegial support and an orientation to the culture of academic medicine; senior faculty, who aid in skill development; and distance mentors, who help to expand the mentee's practical knowledge of the field and his or her professional network.

Other scholars, focusing specifically on AIDS, mental health and illness, and correctional health, have suggested that the creation of partnerships between historically Black colleges and universities (HBCUs) and other research institutions would help to address the relative scarcity of minority physicians and behavioral scientists in high-level research programs with a focus in these areas (Treadwell et al., 2009). Although HBCUs constitute only 3% of the approximately 4,084 institutions of higher education in the United States, they include approximately 14% of all African American students and confer almost 25% of all undergraduate degrees earned by African American students (United States Department of Education, 2010).

Reliance on such alternative models of mentoring may also lead to unanticipated benefits for minority faculty. Minority faculty members are often subject to what has euphemistically been called "cultural taxation" (Padilla, 1994) and "minority faculty syndrome" (Dolcini, Reznick, & Marín, 2009). Because they are members of a minority group, they may be called upon to serve as "experts" on matters of diversity, although they may not, in fact, be experts in diversity; to educate others about issues related to diversity; to serve on university committees that address diversity; to serve as a link between the university and minority communities; to negotiate disagreements that may be attributable to misunderstandings stemming form cultural differences; and, for those who speak languages others than English, to translate documents or interpret conversations for others. Minority faculty may feel that they are in a "double bind"; a refusal to provide these services may provoke charges of poor citizenship and threaten their chances for promotion and tenure, while acquiescence to such requests may deprive the faculty member of the time necessary to prepare publishable manuscripts and impede his or her professional advancement (Padilla, 1994; Rabionet, Santiago, & Zorrilla, 2009; Wyatt et al., 2009).

White mentors at HBCUs may also confront issues relating to racial and ethnic diversity. It has been suggested that White faculty who mentor students at HBCUs may be held to a higher standard and may suffer increased scrutiny from their colleagues and students because of the historical legacy that exists between African Americans and Whites in this country (Foster, 2001).

Mentors may avoid discussing issues related to racial/ethnic difference for several reasons. First, they may believe that race/ethnicity should have no bearing on and does not determine one's professional success and achievement (Davidson & Foster-Johnson, 2001). Alternatively, they may be hesitant to raise such issues, fearing that their attention to such issues will provoke accusations of racism. Mentees may be reluctant to discuss issues of race and ethnicity because they are unsure of their own identity and/or are uncertain about the organization's perception of their race or ethnicity (Davidson & Foster-Johnson, 2001; Thomas, 1990).

Numerous suggestions have been offered as strategies for the improvement of cross-race mentoring relationships. Mentors are urged to develop an increased self-understanding and self-awareness with respect to their own professional goals, their professional strengths and weakness, and their attitudes toward racial and ethnic difference (Davidson & Foster-Johnson, 2001). Mentors are encouraged to develop an increased understanding of their mentee with respect to the mentee's ethnic maturity level, strengths and weaknesses, professional goals, values, and difficulties experienced in response to his/her race or ethnicity. It is also important that the mentor understand the perspective of the organization in which the mentoring relationship occurs, as well as the social networks that may be available to the mentee through the organization (Davidson & Foster-Johnson, 2001).

Race, Ethnicity, and Mentoring Junior-Level Professionals

Four barriers to success as a minority researcher in academia have been identified: inadequate research infrastructure, training, and development; obstacles in the development of an independent research career, such as overemployment as a co-investigator; inadequate culturally relevant mentoring; and insensitivity, miscommunications, and misperceptions (Shavers et al., 2005). Minority individuals may also be dissuaded from entering academic medicine or health because of the long legacy that exists in the United States of unethical research that specifically targeted or largely involved minority populations (Arbour & Cook, 2006; Hornblum, 1998; Shafer, 2004; Thomas & Quinn, 1991; Ward, 1936).

Although mentoring programs may play a critical role in the ability of minority faculty to succeed in their academic institutions, participation may be hampered by the institutional environment. Many universities emphasize independence, autonomy, and competitiveness. Consequently, individuals who participate as mentees in a mentoring program may be perceived as, or may fear that they will be perceived as, somehow not good enough and that such perceptions will adversely affect their career progress (Boyle & Boice, 1998; Girves, Zepeda, & Gwathmey, 2005).

Research findings suggest that although mentor race is not a factor in the professional development of African American junior faculty, it is a factor in the ability of the mentee to address feelings of isolation and the mentee's perception of his or her value to the academic department (Tillman, 2001). Only 3% of college and university faculty are African American; African American women are underrepresented to an even greater degree, comprising only 1% of all college faculty (Bowman, Kite, Branscombe, & Williams, 2000; Menges & Exum, 1983). In addition, African American women may be doubly impacted by sexism and racism (Menges & Exum, 1983). As a result of their relative absence from the academy, African American women have been characterized as "isolated, underutilized, and often demoralized" (Carroll, 1973, p. 173).

The isolation and marginalization experienced by some minority faculty may be exacerbated as a result of microaggressions, that is, "the chronic, everyday injustices that people of color endure—the interpersonal and environmental messages that are denigrating, demeaning, or invalidating" (Walters & Simoni, 2009, p. S73). These may take the form of subtle, dismissive microinsults, such as eye-rolling in response to a comment; microinvalidations, exemplified by a minority group's omission in discussion; or microassaults, such as racist comments or jokes aimed at the minority faculty member (Sue et al., 2007).

Flexibility with respect to the mentoring model to be utilized for minority junior faculty may be required. It has been suggested that the classic mentoring model that entails a one-to-one relationship between unequals in knowledge and power, with the corresponding expectation of deference on the part of the mentee, may be perceived by some minority faculty members as paternalistic and racist. Minority faculty members may react negatively, perhaps on an unconscious level, to this structure as a result of their marginalization and disenfranchisement (Margolis & Romero, 2001).

Institutional commitment at the funder level is critical to the development and sustainability of mentoring programs for health researchers from underrepresented minority groups (Forsyth & Stoff, 2009). That commitment must include adequate financial support for training and conferences; support for the formation of partnerships between better-funded institutions and educational institutions that serve primarily minorities; and the collection and analysis of data to monitor and evaluate the rates of recruitment, retention, and promotion of faculty from underrepresented minority groups.

One example of a highly successful mentoring program for faculty involved in behavioral research in health is that of the University of California San Francisco's (UCSF) Visiting Professors Program (Dolcini, Reznick, & Marín, 2009). This program selects each year between three and five visiting professors through a competitive process to participate in a three-year program. As of 2007, approximately 40 research scientists had completed or were enrolled in the program. Components of the program include a summer institute of six weeks' duration over the course of three consecutive summers; institute activities, such as research planning seminars, networking and mentoring meetings, and guest lectures and seminars; summer stipends to support the visiting professors; seed funds for the conduct of preliminary research studies; a commitment from the professors' home institutions of a minimum of 25% protected time for research activities; the facilitation of professional networking; and one-on-one mentoring with a selected mentor during the course of the year. Training is provided in the areas of grant development, research design and data analysis, and manuscript preparation. Because the summer institutes occur over three consecutive years, they include both current and past cohorts of visiting professors, thereby facilitating the development of professional networks between the mentees.

Minority health professionals may continue to experience a sense of isolation and marginalization even after their entry into the clinical workforce (Duchscher & Cowin, 2004). A study involving 17 Latina nursing students in Connecticut and Massachusetts found that the nurses often felt marginalized because of their ethnicity and pressure to assimilate (Rivera-Goba & Nieto, 2007). Mentoring has been held to be essential to the ability of African American nurses to navigate successfully through our current health care system (Giger & Davidhizar, 1993).

Race, Ethnicity, and Organizational-Structural Considerations

Davidson and Foster-Johnson (2001) have suggested that the organizational culture may play a large role in the success or failure of a minority student. They have decried the assumption by a majority of graduate schools that minority students will assimilate into the dominant organizational, social, and economic culture by adopting the behaviors and values of that dominant organizational culture. Such a perspective both ignores "the structural process of institutional racism, power, and identity" in relation to those who are expected to assimilate and devalues alternative cultural and racial experiences (Cropper, 2000, p. 599). Other scholars have similarly argued that a mentoring focus on the individual and a failure to address structural issues only serves to maintain the status quo (Gulam and Zulfiqar, 1998; cf. Daly & Lumley, 2008). The result may be a sense of marginalization on the part of the minority students (Preece, 1999).

Davidson and Foster-Johnson (2001) advocate instead that graduate programs adopt a perspective of cultural pluralism that recognizes the diversity of the students' cultural backgrounds and the contributions of each student to the culture of the graduate school. They note that the unwillingness of many graduate schools to address issues of culture, race, and ethnicity in course work outside of the social sciences is a disservice to all students, not only URM students; the incorporation of such issues in course work would train students to examine problems and issues from multiple perspectives across disciplinary domains.

Mentoring programs and the institutions in which they reside have been further criticized for their failure to recognize and address the cultural differences that may exist between URM students and others, and the implications of such differences on student expectations and performance (Davidson & Foster-Johnson, 2001). Individuals from the nondominant culture may utilize communication styles that differ from that of the dominant culture; these differences may lead to erroneous assumptions and misunderstandings. Individuals from cultures that value expressiveness may be viewed by those within the dominant culture as histrionic. Medical school students whose cultures stress cooperation rather than competition may find it difficult to be assertive during rounds, leading other to draw faulty conclusions, such as the students' inability to adapt to medical culture (Abernethy, 1999).

Related to communication style, individuals from diverse cultures may utilize methods of dealing with and resolving conflict that differ from those of the dominant culture (Davidson & Foster-Johnson, 2001). Such differences may also give rise to faulty assumptions and misunderstandings. As an example, individuals from an ethnic community that values forthrightness above harmony may be perceived as aggressive or antagonistic in their attempts to address conflict directly.

Whether faculty view cross-race mentoring as a priority or see it as an option may largely depend on the organizational environment (Barker, 2007). The extent to which financial and staff resources are committed to support mentoring in general and to address issues of diversity specifically sends a strong message to both faculty and students (Cropper, 2000). The implementation of formal departmental-level events to examine, discuss, and address issues related to diversity can serve as a signal of encouragement to both mentors and mentees in cross-cultural mentoring relationships to address issues of racial and ethnic diversity. Other departmental-level activities that may lay the foundation for a more welcoming environment and foster effective cross-race mentoring relationships include requiring diversity training; developing and implementing systems to monitor the occurrence and resolution of diversity issues, to facilitate students' ability to express diversity-related concerns (Davidson & Foster-Johnson, 2001); and encouraging collaborations on research endeavors that incorporate issues of race or ethnicity and utilization of a variety of teaching approaches to address diversity issues.

One example of an environment conducive to discussing issues of diversity generally and race specifically is that created by the Medical Student Mentoring Program at the University of Rochester School of Medicine (Abernethy, 1999). That mentoring program, which was funded by the New York State Department of Health, sought to address the needs of underrepresented minority students as they progressed through their training. Mentors were selected based on recommendations of minority and nonminority faculty, minority students, and the Office of Ethnic and Multicultural Affairs. Prospective mentors were advised that the program had the support of the associate dean. Mentee discussion at reflection group meetings, which were facilitated by a clinical psychologist, included handling racially biased encounters, maintaining a bicultural perspective, and conflict resolution strategies. Mentor training included a focus on lack of awareness of cultural biases, faculty discomfort with differentness, and strategies for resolving conflict. The minority mentees, all of whom were paired with nonminority mentors, indicated that they had been able to discuss racial issues with their mentors; the students identified their mentors' openness and honesty as critical to this process.

CONSIDERATIONS OF SEX, GENDER ROLE, AND SEXUAL ORIENTATION

Similar to the corporate world in which there are relatively few women at the highest leadership levels (Catalyst, 1996), there are relatively few women at the highest ranks of academia, despite the growing numbers of women entering the health professions (Health Resources and Services

Administration, 1995; Nonnemaker, 2000). This relative absence of women at the highest levels of academia translates into a lack of role models and mentors for women and may constitute a major barrier to the advancement of women in their careers (Mark et al., 2001). This is true, for example, in academic medicine (Nonnemaker, 2000), graduate departments of psychology (Russo, Olmedo, Stapp, & Fulcher, 1981), and social work education (Holley & Young, 2005; McPhail, 2004). As of 1985, only 10% of female medical school faculty held the rank of full professor (Bickel et al., 2002). This had increased to only 12% by as recently as 2006 (Magrane, Lang, & Alexander, 2006). In contrast, 30% of male faculty held the rank of full professor for the past two decades (Bickel et al., 2002). Female applicants for academic positions in psychology are often perceived as less competent than their male counterparts with identical credentials and are consequently less likely to be considered for the position (Steinpreis, Anders, & Ritzke, 1999). Although women constitute a numerical majority of those involved in social work education, they are less likely than men, including men of color, to hold administrative positions or tenure (Holley & Young, 2005; McPhail, 2004).

Research findings indicate that women in academia may prefer to be mentored by other women. In part, this may be attributable to a desire for a mentor who can demonstrate the ability to balance work and family obligations (Bruce, 1995; Clark & Corcoran, 1986). However, it appears both that women are less likely to be available as mentors and, when they are, may not address this mentoring need (Simon, Roff, & Perry, 2008).

As indicated, the relative unavailability of female mentors may be attributable, at least in part, to the scarcity of women in the highest ranks of academia (Ragins, 1997). This may be particularly true in academic medicine, despite the increasing numbers of women in medical school (Levinson, Kaufman, Clark, & Tolle, 1991; Mark et al., 2001). This scarcity of high-ranking women faculty, together with the attainment by more men of higher rank within organizations, including health care organizations (Koberg, Bosos, & Goodman, 1998), has resulted in an increased likelihood that women in many health professions will have a male mentor and that those women who are available as mentors will shoulder a disproportionately large share of the mentoring responsibilities. For example, 44% of medical students at one institution reported that they had a female mentor, but women represented only 24% of the faculty (Aagaard & Hauer, 2003). Additionally, women at mid-career levels may be reluctant to take on mentees, feeling that the "glass ceiling" limits both their ability to move forward on their career trajectory and their ability to mentor others (Russell, 1994).

A number of studies suggest, however, that men and women are more likely to select a male mentor when offered a choice. Erkut and Mokros (1984) reported that male college students were less likely to select a female mentor because they perceived women as having less power than men. In another study involving 89 female psychologists, the investigator reported that male mentors were perceived as having greater power than their female counterparts (Brefach, 1986).

Research findings relating to the effects of cross-sex mentorship outside of the health professions has yielded inconsistent findings. Mentorship by male mentors has been found to be associated with greater compensation (Dreher & Cox, 1996; Wallace, 2001) and increased career development functions (Sosik & Godshalk, 2000) compared to mentorship by either female or minority mentors. Although a number of studies have reported that women receive greater psychosocial support and role modeling from female mentors (Burke, McKeen, & McKenna, 1990; Sosik & Godshalk, 2000; Thomas, 1990), others have found no such differences (Ragins and McFarlin, 1990). Scandura and Ragins (1993) observed that individuals having an androgynous sex role orientation reported receiving more mentoring functions in comparison with their counterparts with masculine or feminine role orientations. Research on cross-sex mentoring indicates that the mentoring experience may be marred by paternalism, overprotection, and/or sexual tension (Kram, 1985; Noe, 1988a, 1988b; Ragins & Cotton, 1991).

Relatively little research has been conducted relating to mentoring lesbian, gay, bisexual, transgender, and questioning (LGBTQ) students and professionals in health-related careers. Research relating to workplace environments in general suggests that concerns include the impact of heterosexism, homophobia, and discrimination on career advancement and job satisfaction (Croteau, 1996; Lyons, Brenner, & Fassinger, 2005; Morrow, Gore, & Campbell, 1996; Nauta, Saucier, & Woodard, 2001).

Sex, Gender Role, and Sexual Orientation: Mentoring Students

There is evidence to suggest both that female students face difficulty in identifying appropriate female mentors and that structural issues may limit their ability to identify and work with any mentor. Research conducted with women in departments of psychology have found that, compared with their male counterparts, women receive a smaller share of nonfederal aid and smaller financial awards (Solomon, 1978; Syverson, 1982), are less likely to receive funding that involves working with a faculty member on research, are more likely to be given teaching assistantships in lieu of research assistantships, and are more likely to rely on their own financial resources to fund their graduate education (Solomon, 1976). It has been suggested that women's reduced opportunity to receive funding that is associated with research ultimately impairs their ability to develop a mentor–mentee relationship (Rogat & Redner, 1985). Male mentors may be reluctant to take on women as mentees for fear that their colleagues will attribute unethical motives to them (Johnson & Huwe, 2002).

Whether women reap the same level of benefits from a mentoring relationship as men remains somewhat unclear. An early study found that female mentees in psychology were less likely to be offered opportunities to accompany a professor on a professional trip, to meet scholars in other departments, or to be credited with authorship in conjunction with their research participation (O'Connell et al., 1978). However, more recent studies suggest that when women are able to obtain mentoring, male mentors are equally as likely as female mentors to encourage their graduate female psychology students to conduct research and to provide the students with appropriate opportunities to do so (Dohm & Cummings, 2002; Hollingsworth & Fassinger, 2002). These differences in research findings may be attributable to characteristics of the particular study samples and the sampling strategy, the study design, and/or to changes during the intervening years in mentoring approaches in graduate psychology programs.

Lesbian, gay, bisexual, transgender, and questioning (LGBTQ) students may also encounter difficulties in identifying a suitable mentor. Research findings indicate that LGBTQ graduate students are often concerned about the response that they will receive if they make their sexual orientation known ("come out") and whether their ability to obtain work or funding will be adversely impacted as a result (Lark & Croteau, 1998). LGBTQ students have been found to consider the availability of support for LGBTQ-related issues in making decisions about graduate programs, to prefer mentors with a similar sexual orientation who are knowledgeable about LGBTQ-related issues (Lark & Croteau, 1998; McAllister, Ahmedani, Harold, & Cramer, 2009), and to perceive greater support from lesbian and gay mentors as compared with heterosexual mentors (Lin, 2001).

The mentor's prestige may be a significant factor in the mentee's career trajectory. A study of male biochemists found that the mentor's citation record was associated with the mentee's first academic appointment and the number of publications that the mentee achieved during the first three years following completion of his doctoral degree (Long, 1978). These data suggest that the mentor's level of expertise and achievement in research may contribute significantly to a mentee's development of the skills necessary for professional success.

Sex, Gender Role, and Sexual Orientation: Mentoring Junior-Level Professionals

The importance of a mentor for junior faculty in the health sciences cannot be overstated. In academic medicine, there exists a significant association between having a mentor and time spent in research, the number of publications, and overall career satisfaction (Levinson et al., 1991). Male faculty may be assigned tasks or committees carrying higher prestige, thereby providing them with greater access to higher status persons than their female counterparts; this access may increase the ability of male faculty to develop larger professional networks that comprise individuals of higher status (Robinson, 1973). Investigators conducting a survey of academic medical school faculty found that men were more likely than their female counterparts to report that their mentors had facilitated their external visibility through activities such as inviting them to chair a conference session or offering them authorship on a publication (Fried et al., 1996). In contrast, female faculties participating in the survey were more likely to indicate that the mentor had utilized the mentee's work to benefit their own careers. A later study similarly found that female faculties were less likely to be invited to participate in informal networking events than were their male colleagues (Palepu et al., 1998).

Several similarities between the situation confronting minority faculty and that confronting women faculty are notable. Like minority faculty, women faculty may encounter various forms of hostility, unfairness, and inappropriateness in the work environment that does not rise to the level of discrimination as it is defined by law. These behaviors, which have been termed "microinequities" (Rowe, 1990), include *supportive discouragement*; *collegial exclusion* ("forgetting" to invite a female colleague to a lunch or dinner meeting); *radiant devaluation* ("You're much too petite and courteous to be in emergency medicine"); *friendly harassment* ("I know how important your family is; I wouldn't want you to tear yourself away for this meeting"); *benevolent exploitation* ("Why don't you take on teaching this other course; it will protect your time from others' demands"); and *considerate domination* ("I'm only telling you to teach this course to protect you from other pressures") (Lenhart & Evans, 1991).

As with minority faculty, it has been suggested that the classic dyadic model of mentoring is inadequate to address the needs of women faculty members. This may be particularly true in academic medicine, due to the lack of many senior women faculty (Mayer, Blair, & Files, 2006). In addition, although male mentors may be effective as career mentors for women in medicine, they are less likely than female mentors to provide personal advice. Accordingly, scholars have recommended that women in medicine (1) identify a mentor of either sex to provide career mentoring and a second female mentor to provide guidance with respect to a work-family balance; and/or (2) utilize a network of peers for mentoring (Levinson et al., 1991).

Women in clinical practice may face similar difficulties. A study involving 271 female physicians in rural practice in Australia found that they face a number of issues that could be ameliorated with mentoring by more senior female physicians (Wainer, 2004). These include the lack of ongoing adequate skill development, the relative lack of support from male colleagues, the lack of flexibility in professional practice, and difficulties balancing family and career obligations. Although the study was conducted in Australia, it is likely that many of these same issues are confronted by female physicians practicing in rural areas of the United States.

Sex, Gender Role, and Sexual Orientation: Organizational and Structural Considerations

When a group with a specific characteristic comprises 20% or less than the larger group, the group is said to be "skewed" and those displaying the discrepant characteristic—in this case, being female or nonheterosexual—may become the focus of unwarranted attention (Kanter, 1977). This may take the form of microinequities, as described above, or may manifest in other forms in the organization.

Additionally, numerous structural barriers exist that impede women's ability to move forward on their career trajectories. Often, attainment of tenure for faculty in a medical school requires a work week of 60 or more hours. However, only about one-third of medical schools have policies relating to maternity leave that go beyond its categorization as disability leave; less than one-quarter have child care facilities (Grisso, Hansen, Zellinq, Bickel, & Eisenberg, 1991). Part-time faculty may not be entitled to fringe benefits and may be expected to work longer hours than they are actually paid for. Women who work less than full-time are often perceived as lacking commitment to their careers and are dismissed (Bickel, 1995). Not surprisingly, several surveys of women physicians have indicated that competing work and family demands constitute a major contributor to career dissatisfaction and adversely impact physicians' career aspirations (Mayer et al., 2006).

Alternative Models of Mentoring for Women

It has been suggested that the traditional model of mentoring, which is hierarchical in style and emphasizes independence and competition (Colley, 2000; Johnson-Bailey & Cervero, 2002) rather than interpersonal relationships and collaboration, may not be the best approach for mentoring women. Scholars have also noted that the traditional model of mentoring is paternalistic, is premised on a model of male career development, and assumes that one style of mentoring is adequate to meet the needs of all mentees (Benishek, Bieschke, Paryk, & Slattery, 2004). A variety of other models have been proffered as potentially more suitable for women. These include the multiple mentor model, peer mentoring, and the multicultural feminist model of mentoring.

In contrast to the traditional model, the multiple mentor model can include both senior- and junior-level faculty members or colleagues, thereby providing an opportunity for both collaborative and hierarchical relationships. Multiple mentors may also offer increased opportunities for professional networking.

Peer mentoring offers some of the same advantages as does the multiple mentor model, such as psychosocial support and the advantages that attach to having multiple mentors. This model, which has been utilized in the context of academic medicine (Pololi & Knight, 2005; Pololi, Knight, Dennis, & Frankel, 2002), permits greater flexibility than the traditional model of mentoring and may allow women to balance more easily the demands of their professional and personal lives (Limbert, 1995; Pololi et al., 2002). However, it may not be an effective mechanism for mentoring if all of the members of the group are equally inexperienced.

The multicultural feminist model of mentoring (Benishek et al., 2004) is derived from the feminist mentoring model (Fassinger, 1997). The feminist model is premised on the recognition and acknowledgement of the power differential that exists between the mentor and the mentee and proposes that the mentor's power be utilized as a means of empowering the mentee. The multicultural feminist model (MFM) expands upon this by suggesting that the mentor assume responsibility for (1) raising multicultural issues with all mentees, (2) encouraging mentees to seek out additional mentors and to develop a "constellation of mentors" (Benishek et al., 2004, p. 437), and (3) welcoming diverse perspectives. As such, the model recognizes that education and science are not value-free. The MFM also requires that the mentor and the mentee examine explicitly differences in power and privilege (Benishek et al., 2004).

Each of these alternative approaches to mentoring may be important not only for women, but also for individuals who self-identify as gay, lesbian, bisexual, or transgender. Individuals who self-identify as such may be reluctant to express their concerns to a single mentor, who may not offer a safe environment in which to do so. The development of a mentoring network that includes multiple individuals, whether through a multiple mentor model, a larger peer mentoring network, or the MFM model, increases the likelihood that an individual who self-identifies as nonheterosexual will be able to locate one or more suitable mentors (Benishek et al., 2004).

MENTORING IN THE INTERNATIONAL CONTEXT

As indicated above, increasing proportions of students and practitioners in health care professions in the United States are not U.S. citizens, and have come to the United States to further their training and/or to practice their profession. In addition to the issues that confront minority and female students and professionals in health-related careers, international health students and professionals may encounter other issues directly attributable to the international experience and their repatriation upon their return to their home countries. The specific issues vary across the various stages of the international experience, described below.

Stages of the International Experience

Crocitto, Sullivan, and Carraher (2006) have suggested that international mentees, or newcomers, progress through multiple learning cycles as they strive to accomplish their tasks in the host country. Each cycle consists of four stages: exploration, trial, establishment, and mastery. The beginning of the learning cycle occurs predeparture, while the newcomer is still in the country of his or her last residence and is making preparations for the new experience. The most intense part of this learning cycle occurs during the expatriation stage, when the mentee is on-site in the host country. The final phase occurs during the repatriation stage, when the newcomer is repatriated into his or her home country.

International mentees to the United States may be at high risk of failure due to a lack of cultural awareness and an inability to adapt to their new environment (Crocitto, Sullivan, & Carraher, 2006). It has been suggested that the likelihood of success could be increased if linkages were maintained with the home country during the on-site phase of the learning cycle and if the expatriates were to have several concurrent mentors who together could address the mentee's varied developmental needs (Mezias & Scandura, 2005). As an example, the mentee will need information about the receiving country, the culture of both the receiving country and the organization in which the mentee will be functioning, and the expectations of the mentee in the new location. Reliance on a multiple mentor model may be the most effective approach to assist the mentee with his or her physical or psychological transitions (Crocitto et al., 2006; de Janasz & Sullivan, 2004).

Unfortunately, relatively little international mentoring exists throughout the various cycles of an international mentee's experience. This has been attributed to several factors including the complex nature of international mentoring, individuals' tendency to overestimate the cost of such a relationship relative to the benefits (Ragins & Scandura, 1999), the physical distance involved, and the absence of organizational rewards for participating in such mentoring arrangements (Crocitto et al., 2006).

Mentoring During the Predeparture Stage

Crocitto et al. (2006) have identified four critical functions to be accomplished by the mentee during the predeparture stage: (1) the identification of knowledgeable mentors; (2) an assessment of the potential impact of the international move on his or her career trajectory; (3) the identification of and response to family concerns regarding the international move; and (4) the development of a relationship with an individual who will serve as a "relocation mentor," keeping the mentee informed about relevant events in the home country while he or she is overseas. The selection of a relocation mentor is particularly critical; this individual bears responsibility for assisting the mentee in locating suitable employment following his or her return to the home country.

Mentoring During the Expatriation Stage

It is not unusual for international students and professionals to experience culture shock upon their arrival in the United States. The term "culture shock" was utilized by Kalvero Oberg in 1954 to refer to an "abrupt loss of the familiar" or the "shock of the new." It

> is precipitated by the anxiety that results from losing all familiar signs and symbols of social intercourse. These signs are the thousand and one ways in which we orient ourselves to the situations of daily life: when to shake hands, when and how to be gracious and appropriate . . . when to accept invitations, how to take statements seriously . . . . (Oberg, 1954, p. 1)

As a result, individuals may experience feelings of inadequacy, vulnerability, anger, resentment, and irritability, and find that they are unable to solve even simple problems because of their lack of familiarity with the new environment. As a result, they may lack self-confidence and have a tendency to blame others for any difficulties.

Culture shock occurs in various stages or phases, which have been variously termed incubation, crisis, recovery, and full recovery (Oberg, 1954, 1960); elation, depression, recovery, and acculturation (Richardson, 1974); and contact, disintegration, reintegration, autonomy, and independence (Adler, 1975). The features of the various phases are similar across these taxonomies. The first stage is characterized by feelings of excitement, which may last for hours, days, weeks, or months. These feelings gradually dissipate, as the individual becomes increasingly aware of the differences that exist between her previous and current environments. This second phase is marked by practical problems, an increase in misunderstandings and associated feelings of frustration, a sense of loneliness and uneasiness, and a decrease in self-confidence. During the third stage of culture shock, the individual will begin to reintegrate into the new environment or reject her new situation, blaming others, and adopting negative coping mechanisms, such as substance use and self-isolation. During the final stage, the individual may gradually adjust and adapt to the new environment, experiencing a greater sense of control, autonomy, and belonging.

Significant variation exists between individuals in their experience of culture shock. The sequence and rate through which they pass through the various stages may differ as a function of their mental state, personality, familiarity with language, family and social support system, religious beliefs, level of education, socioeconomic condition, sex and gender, and past experiences with travel.

International students and professionals may experience difficulties in socialization during their residence in the United States. Social support networks may be critical to the ability of international students to cope with academic stress (Wan, Chapman, & Biggs, 1992). Research suggests that international mentees who are successful in the socialization process are more likely to express satisfaction with their experience and to complete their overseas tasks (Black, 1992; Mendenhall & Oddon, 1985).

Mentoring may also play a critical role in assisting mentees with both socialization to the group and socialization to the task. Socialization to the group refers to the extent to which the newcomers are comfortable with their peers and group norms. International mentees may experience difficulty socializing to the group because host-country nationals may be less open to those from another culture or country than they are to those of the host country. In essence, the international mentee must break through what has been termed an inclusionary boundary (Schein, 1971). The mentor can assist the mentee in his or her efforts to transition from being an outsider to being an included colleague by orienting the mentee to the new environment, providing useful advice, and spending time with the mentee. These efforts on the part of the mentor may help to reduce the mentee's levels of insecurity and uncertainty, and increase his or her comfort level in the organization (Chatman, 1991; Feldman, 1976; Heimann & Pittenger, 1996; Morrison, 1993; Ostroff & Kozlowski, 1993).

Socialization to the task refers to the extent to which the newcomers understand organizational procedures and can perform their responsibilities (Chao, O'Leary-Kelly, Wolf, Klein, & Gardner, 1994; Feldman, 1976; Van Maanen & Schein, 1979). It has been suggested that international graduate students may be less likely than those from the United States to subscribe to traditional scientific norms (Anderson & Louis, 1994).

However, many international students may experience significant difficulties in establishing a mentor–mentee relationship in their new country because of their lack of adequate language skills (Wan et al., 1992). This creates a double-bind for them, because they may realize that a mentoring relationship is necessary in order for them to develop better language skills. Difficulties in communication may be exacerbated by well-intentioned, but ill-advised efforts by instructors to reduce the level of language used with international students, thereby reducing students' opportunity to become more proficient in their use of the host country language (Hellstén & Prescott, 2004).

Additional mechanisms have been proposed to assist international students in their efforts to adjust to the culture of both the host country and the academic institution. These include a course online bulletin board, through which international students can interact with other students (Bellis & Clarke, 2001); the development of bridging programs to assist international students in their transition process (Ryan, 2000); and the development of mentoring programs to address specifically the needs of international students (Crocitto et al., 2006). Four elements are necessary for a cross-cultural mentoring program to be effective. The mentor must have (1) knowledge and an understanding of the mentee's culture; (2) a "flexible cultural lens"; (3) good communication skills; and (4) a desire to understand how the mentor–mentee relationship is impacted by individuals' cultures (Zachary, 2000).

Mentoring During the Repatriation Stage

During the repatriation stage, the mentee may experience reverse culture shock (Adler, 1981). They may be unaware of changes that have occurred during their absence or may find that their situations in their home country are no longer satisfying (Adler, 1991). According to Crocitto et al. (2006), international mentees must accomplish three tasks during the repatriation stage, two of which are relevant to the mentoring context: (1) assess the knowledge, skills, and abilities that were gained during their experience in the host country; and (2) intensify communication with the home country and the relocation mentor in order to identify potential opportunities, and how best to utilize the international experience following return to the home country.

Following repatriation, mentees can serve as a source of knowledge about the host country's culture and opportunities that may exist there. Because of their experience, they may be particularly helpful to individuals who later travel to the host country by providing them with contacts within their previously developed social networks. The case study by Dr. Beatrice Ioan, which follows this chapter, provides an example of how a mentee can utilize his or her training experience and knowledge gained in the host country to develop a field of endeavor and her own career trajectory upon return to the home country.

BARRIERS TO EFFECTIVE DIVERSIFIED MENTORING

Stereotyping

Stereotyping has been defined as "a cognitive structure that contains the perceiver's knowledge, beliefs, and expectancies about some human group" (Hamilton & Trolier, 1986, p. 133). Stereotypes serve as the basis for the categorization of others into groups; this process helps us make sense of the world around us and gives us some sense of control. However, classifying individuals on the basis of socially constructed categories of race and ethnicity may reinforce racial and ethnic divisions that already exist (Azuonye, 1996; Bogue & Edwards, 1971; Fullilove, 1998; Stolley, 1999) and adversely affect the mentoring relationship.

As an example of how this might occur, consider the concept of competence. It is important to a mentoring relationship that the mentor and the mentee perceive each other as competent. The perception of competence, though, is highly susceptible to stereotypes (Ilgen & Youtz, 1986). One study found, for example, that the success of African American managers was attributed to help from other individuals, rather than to their own ability and effort (Greenhaus & Parasuraman, 1993). A mentor who holds a stereotypical belief relating to the ability of African Americans and applies it uniformly to all African American mentees may perceive a mentee as less capable. This belief, founded on a stereotype of African Americans, may lead to a lack of interest in the mentee's career development and a failure to invest adequate time, energy, and attention in the development of the relationship. A mentee who perceives his or her mentor as less intelligent, and therefore less competent, may become disinterested in his or her work and may fail to recognize opportunities and advantages that are offered by the relationship.

Similarly, women may be perceived to be more emotional, less logical, and less assertive than men, and therefore as less qualified than men to manage or lead (Baumgardner, Lord, & Maher, 1992; Heilman, Block, Martell, & Simon, 1989; Noe, 1988a, 1988b). One highly publicized example of a stereotype-in-action is the statement by then-Harvard University president Lawrence Summers that women's failure to advance in mathematics and science and difficulties in recruiting and retaining women faculty in these disciplines was attributable to "innate" differences in women's and men's abilities (Lawler, 2005).

International students and health professionals may similarly be the targets of perceptions and behaviors that are rooted in stereotypes (Ninnes, Aitchison, & Kalos, 1999; Spencer-Rodgers & McGovern, 2002). A comprehensive study of students' attitudes toward their international peers found that the U.S. students often characterized their foreign classmates as frightened, sad, lonely, and depressed (Spencer-Rodgers & McGovern, 2002). Respondents also reported feeling uncomfortable, impatient, and frustrated when having to communicate with foreign students. Graduate students, in particular, expressed the belief that foreign students were utilizing an unfair share of educational resources. International students who are perceived to have English language deficits may be subject to particularly derogatory evaluation by their peers (Spencer-Rodgers, 2001). Although undergraduate students have evaluated international students performing in the capacity of student-instructors extremely negatively (McCroskey, 1998), the perceived level of accentedness, rather than the actual level of accentedness, may be tied to such negative evaluation (Rubin & Smith, 1990).

Individuals who are members of the majority group may also be subject to stereotypes that can negatively impact the formation of productive mentor–mentee relationships. As an example, this author was informed by an international mentee attending a university in a large urban area that she was transferring to another university where she could study under a foreign-born mentor because U.S.-born mentors "all exploit their students." However, when asked if she had had such an experience or knew of someone who had experienced such a situation, she replied that she had not, but that a transfer would prevent such a situation from ever arising.

The application of a stereotype to all individuals perceived to be members of a particular category of persons is known as category-based responding (Miller & Brewer, 1986). The category provides the basis for distinguishing between individuals who are deemed by the observer to be members of the "in-group" and those who are to be considered part of the "out-group." Differentiated responding is somewhat less rigid. Although distinctions are still drawn between those in the in-group and those in the out-group on the basis of the observer's categorization, distinctions are made between members of the in-group. Personalized responding is the least rigid approach, involving the least stereotyping, to distinguishing those in the in- and out-groups. Individuals using this approach respond to others on the basis of their individual characteristics and qualities, rather than on the basis of perceived group characteristics and predetermined socially constructed categories and expectations (Miller & Brewer, 1986).

Accordingly, it is critical that mentors develop an awareness of their own preconceptualizations and the stereotypes and biases that exist within the larger context in which the mentor–mentee relationship is situated. This self-awareness and a willingness and openness to discuss with mentees their observations and experiences of bias may be critical to the establishment of rapport and trust between the mentor and the mentee. Such discussions require sensitivity and empathy, so as not to be construed by the mentee as a diminution of his or her competence or an attribution of fault. Such discussions also require self-awareness, willingness, and openness on the part of the mentee.

Discrimination

Scholars have cautioned that the support of informal mentoring efforts or the implementation of formal mentoring programs without prior thought as to their impact on the workforce is fraught with legal hazards

(Harshman & Rudin, 2001). They have suggested that even well-intentioned programs may inadvertently result in disparate impact or disparate treatment for members of protected legal groups, in violation of the provisions of Title VII of the Civil Rights Act of 1964.

For example, an organization, such as a university, might provide support for an informal mentoring program through publicity, allocation of faculty salary for mentoring junior faculty, and a small budget to support informal mentoring activities. The self-selection process whereby the mentors and mentees gravitate toward each other based on perceived similarities and mutual affinity has the potential to perpetuate the status quo. A study involving close to 100 mentors involved in informal mentoring programs found that mentors tend to perceive their protégés as more similar to themselves than are other individuals who are under their direct supervision (Burke, McKenna, & McKeen, 1991). In some cases, depending on the culture of the organization, this could result in the further entrenchment of "good old boy" networks (Mehri, 1997). Research conducted in the corporate context has demonstrated that such informal mentoring schemes can disparately impact men and women, so that women have less access to the highest-ranking members of the company (Viator & Scandura, 1991).

A claim of disparate impact may arise not only from the conduct of the program, but also from the mentoring relationship itself. In *Jensvold v. Shalala* (1993), Margaret Jensvold argued that the differences between her mentoring program and that of her male counterparts were relevant to support her claim that she had been discriminated on the basis of sex, thereby successfully defending against the dismissal of her case.

Institutions can minimize the risk of liability associated with informal training programs through careful examination and monitoring of career pathways and outcomes within the organization. In the context of a formal mentoring program, the likelihood of legal issues arising can be reduced through the development of clearly defined, objective criteria for mentor and mentee participation in the program; consistent adherence to the selection criteria for mentors and mentees by all involved in the selection process; uniform training of all mentors; and documentation of all such efforts and selections (Harshman & Rudin, 2001).

Sexual Harassment

One of the most recognized issues that is raised in conjunction with cross-sex mentoring is the possibility of romantic or sexual involvement between the mentor and the mentee or the perception of such involvement by others in the institution (Blake, 1998; Clawson & Kram, 1984; Devine & Markiewicz, 1990). Women may be unwilling to approach a male for mentorship for fear her request will be misconstrued as a sexual advance (Ragins & Cotton, 1991). Men may similarly be unwilling to mentor a female out of concern that their motives will be misconstrued. There has been growing recognition, however, that romantic/sexual relationships may also occur in the context of same-sex mentor–mentee relationships and that these relationships may give rise to similar legal and ethical issues as cross-sex mentoring relationships.

If a sexual or romantic relationship is initiated between the mentor and the mentee, its later termination may lead to charges of sexual harassment, for example, an implicit or explicit demand for sexual favors in exchange for favorable recommendations, access to important professional opportunities, and so on. The simplest approach to prevent both such accusations and the accompanying emotional pain and professional embarrassment is for the mentor and the mentee to avoid becoming romantically or sexually involved. On a programmatic and organizational level, it should be recognized that the formation of such relationships is a possibility and appropriate procedures developed to manage the relationships if they do occur. For example, many universities have established procedures that permit the reassignment of supervisory responsibilities to another individual in situations in which a supervisor and supervisee become romantically involved. In the context of a mentor–mentee relationship that develops sexually or romantically, responsibility for mentoring should be shifted to one or more other individuals.

SUMMARY

Despite the benefits that have been associated with mentoring, minority individuals—defined broadly to include those whose minority status is attributable to their nationality, race, ethnicity, gender, sex, gender role, sexual orientation, and/or religion—continue to experience difficulty in securing mentoring. Even when mentoring is available, it more likely than not will be with a nonminority mentor. It may consequently be difficult for the mentor or mentee to raise issues related to their differentness and its effects on their mentoring relationship.

Issues of group membership and individual identity are both complex and sensitive. The impact of "differentness," however it is defined, on the mentee experience and professional growth can only be understood in the historical and social context in which group membership is claimed and the relationship occurs. A discussion of such issues between the mentor and the mentee requires that both develop an awareness of the stereotypes that they bring to their interaction and the social, historical, and political context in which their interactions occur. Frankness and honesty in the exploration of these issues may engender new understandings for both the mentor and the mentee.

REFERENCES

Aagaard, E. M., & Hauer, K. E. (2003). A cross-sectional descriptive study of mentoring relationships formed by medical students. *Journal of General Internal Medicine, 18,* 298–302.

Abernethy, A. D. (1999). A mentoring program for underrepresented-minority students at the University of Rochester School of medicine. *Academic Medicine, 74*(4), 356–359.

Adler, N. J. (1981). Re-entry: Managing cross-cultural transitions. *Group and Organizational Studies, 6*(3), 341–356.

Adler, N. J. (1991). *International dimensions of organizational behavior.* Boston, MA: PWS-Kent Publishing Company.

Adler, P. S. (1975). The transitional experience: An alternative view of culture shock. *Journal of Humanistic Psychology, 15*(4), 13–23.

American Association of Colleges of Nursing. (2010). *Nursing shortage fact sheet.* Retrieved May 24, 2010, from http://www.aacn.nche.edu/media/pdf/NrsgShortageFS.pdf

American Council of Education. (2006). *Students of color make dramatic gains in college enrollment but still trail whites in the rate at which they attend college.* Retrieved May 24, 2010, from http://www.acenet.edu/AM/Template.cfm?Section=Publications_and_Products&Contentid=18725&Template=/cm/htmldisplay.cfm.

American Speech-Language-Hearing Association. (2010). *Highlights and trends: ASHA counts for year end 2009.* Retrieved May 29, 2010, from http://www.asha.org/uploadedFiles/2009MemberCounts.pdf

Anderson, M. S., & Louis, K. S. (1994). The graduate student experience and subscription to the norms of science. *Research in Higher Education, 35,* 273–299.

Arbour, L., & Cook, D. (2006). DNA on loan—Issues to consider when carrying out genetic research with aboriginal families and communities. *Community Genetics, 9,* 153–160.

Atkinson, D. R., Neville, H., & Casa, A. (1991). The mentorship of ethnic minorities in professional psychology. *Professional Psychology: Research and Practice, 22,* 336–338.

Azuonye, I. O. (1996). Guidelines will encourage the thinking that underpins racism in medicine. *British Medical Journal, 313,* 426.

Bach, P. B. (2003). Unequal treatment: Confronting racial and ethnic disparities in health care. *New England Journal of Medicine, 349,* 1296–1297.

Barker, M. J. (2007). Cross-cultural mentoring in institutional contexts. *The Negro Educational Review, 58*(1–2), 85–103.

Baumgardner, T. L., Lord, R., & Maher, K. J. (1991). Perceptions of women in management. In R. G. Lord & K. J. Maher (Eds.), *Leadership and information processing: Linking perceptions and performance* (pp. 95–113). Boston, MA: Unwin Hyman.

Bellis, C., & Clarke, S. (Eds.). (2001). *Teaching actuarial management internationally, using the internet.* Sydney, Australia: Centre for Professional Development, Macquairie University. Cited in Crocitto, M. M., Sullivan, S. E., & Carraher, S. M. (2006).

Global mentoring as a means of career development and knowledge creation: A learning-based framework and agenda for future research. *Career Development International, 10*(6/7), 522–535.

Benishek, L. A., Bieschke, K. J., Park, J., & Slattery, S. M. (2004). A multicultural feminist model of mentoring. *Journal of Multicultural Counseling and Development, 32,* 428–442.

Bickel, J. (1995). Scenarios for success—Enhancing women physicians' professional advancement. *Western Journal of Medicine, 162,* 165–169.

Bickel, J., Wara, D., Atkinson, B. F., Cohen, L. S., Dunn, M., Hostler, S., et al. (2002). Association of American Medical Colleges Project Implementation Committee: Increasing women's leadership in academic medicine: Report of the AAMC Project Implementation Committee. *Academic Medicine, 77*(10), 1043–1061.

Black, J. S. (1992). Socializing American expatriate managers overseas. *Group and Organization Management, 17,* 171–192.

Blake, S. D. (1998). An investigation of cross-gender mentoring: Lessons from Harvard University Graduate School of Education's Urban Superintendent Program. In H. T. Frierson (Ed.), *Diversity in higher education, vol. 2: Examining mentor-protégé experiences.* Greenwich, CT: JAI Press.

Bogat, G. A., & Redner, R. L. (1985). How mentoring affects the professional development of women in psychology. *Professional Psychology: Research and Practice, 16*(6), 851–859.

Bogue, G., & Edwards, G. F. (1971). How to get along without race in demographic analysis. *Social Biology, 18,* 387–396.

Bowman, S. R., Kite, M. E., Branscombe, N. R., & Williams, S. (2000). Developmental relationships of Black Americans in the academy. In A. J. Murrell, F. J. Crosby, & R. J. Ely (Eds.), *Mentoring dilemmas: Developmental relationships within multicultural organizations.* Mahwah, NJ: Erlbaum.

Boyle, P., & Boice, B. (1998). Systematic mentoring for new faculty teachers and graduate teaching assistants. *Innovative Higher Education, 22,* 157–179.

Brefach, S. M. (1986). *The mentor experience: The influences of female/male mentors on the personal and professional growth of female psychologists.* Unpublished doctoral dissertation, Boston University, Boston, MA. Cited in O'Neill, R. M., & Blake-Beard, S. D. (2002). Gender barriers to the female mentor-male protégé relationship. *Journal of Business Ethics, 37,* 51–63.

Bruce, M. A. (1995). Mentoring women doctoral students: What counselor educators and supervisors can do. *Counselor Education and Supervision, 35,* 139–149.

Burke, R. J., McKeen, C. A., & McKenna, C. S. (1990). Sex differences and cross-sex effects on mentoring: Some preliminary data. *Psychological Reports, 67,* 1011–1023.

Burke, R. J., McKenna, C. S., & McKeen, C. A. (1991). How do mentorships differ from typical supervisory relationships? *Psychological Reports, 68,* 459–466.

Campbell, A. R., & Davis, S. M. (1996). Faculty commitment: Retaining minority nursing students in majority institutions. *Journal of Nursing Education, 35,* 298–303.

Carroll, C. M. (1973). Three's a crowd: The dilemma of the Black woman in higher education: A strategy for retaining minority faculty. In A. S. Rossi & A. Calderwood (Eds.), *Academic women on the move*. New York: Russell Sage Foundation.

Catalyst. (1996). *Women in corporate leadership: Programs and prospects*. New York: Author.

Chao, G., O'Leary-Kelly, A., Wolf, S., Klein, K., & Gardner, P. (1994). Organizational socialization: Its content and consequences. *Journal of Applied Psychology, 79*, 730–743.

Chatman, J. A. (1991). Matching people and organizations: Selection and socialization in public accounting firms. *Administrative Science Quarterly, 35*, 459–484.

Clark, S. M., & Corcoran, M. (1986). Perspectives on the professional socialization of women faculty. *Journal of Higher Education, 57*(1), 20–43.

Clawson, J. G., & Kram, K. E. (1984). Managing cross-gender mentoring. *Business Horizons, 27*(3), 22–31.

Colley, H. (2000, September). *Exploring myths of mentor: A rough guide to the history of mentoring from a Marxist feminist perspective*. Paper presented at the British Education Research Association Annual Conference, Cardiff University, Cardigg, UK. Cited in Benishek, L. A., Bieschke, K. J., Park, J., & Slatery, S. M. (2004). A multicultural feminist model of mentoring. *Journal of Multicultural Counseling and Development, 32*, 428–442.

Collins, P. M., Kamya, H. A., & Tourse, R. W. (2001). Questions of racial diversity and mentorship: An empirical exploration. *Social Work, 42*(2), 145–152.

Committee on the Guide to Recruiting and Advancing Women Scientists and Engineers in Academia, Committee on Women in Science, Engineering, National Research Council (2006). *To recruit and advance: Women students and faculty in science and engineering*. Washington, DC: National Academies Press.

Crocitto, M. M., Sullivan, S. E., & Carraher, S. M. (2006). Global mentoring as a means of career development and knowledge creation: A learning-based framework and agenda for future research. *Career Development International, 10*(6/7), 522–535.

Cropper, A. (2000). Mentoring as an inclusive device for the excluded: Black students' experience of a mentoring scheme. *Social Work Education, 19*(6), 597–607.

Croteau, J. M. (1996). Research on the work experiences of lesbian, gay, and bisexual people: An integrative review of methodology and findings. *Journal of Vocational Behavior, 48*, 195–209.

Crowley, S., Fuller, D., Law, W., McKeon, D., & Ramirez, J. J. (2004). Improving the climate in research and scientific training environments for members of underrepresented minorities. *Neuroscientist, 10*, 26–30.

Daly, J., & Lumley, J. (2008). Taking care of early-career public health researchers and practitioners. *Australian and New Zealand Journal of Public Health, 32*(3), 203–204.

D'Augelli, A. R., & Hershberger, S. L. (1993). African American undergraduates on a predominantly White campus: Academic factors, social networks, and campus climate. *Journal of Negro Education, 61*, 67–81.

Davidson, M. N. & Foster-Johnson, L. (2001). Mentoring in the preparation of graduate researchers of color. *Review of Educational Research, 71*(4), 549–574.

de Janasz, S., & Sullivan, S. (2004). Multiple mentoring in academe: Developing the professorial network. *Journal of Vocational Behavior, 64*(2), 268–283.

Devine, I., & Markiewicz, D. (1990). Cross-sex relationship at work and the impact of gender stereotypes. *Journal of Business Ethics, 9*, 333–338.

DiTomaso, N., & Hooijberg, R. (1996). Diversity and the demands of leadership. *Quarterly, 7*, 163–187.

Dohm, F.-A., & Cummings, W. (2002). Research mentoring and women in clinical psychology. *Psychology of Women Quarterly, 26*, 163–167.

Dolcini, M. M., Reznick, O. A. G., & Marín, B. V. (2009). Investments in the future of behavioral science: The University of California, San Francisco, Visiting Professors Program. *American Journal of Public Health, 99*(S1), S43–S47.

Dovlo, D. (2005). Taking more than a fair share? The migration of health professionals from poor to rich countries. *PLoS Medicine, 2(5)*, e109.

Dreher, G. F., & Chargois, J. A. (1998). Gender, mentoring experiences, and salary attainment among graduates of an historically Black university. *Journal of Vocational Behavior, 53*, 401–416.

Dreher, G. F., & Cox, T. H. (1996). Race, gender, and opportunity: A study of compensation attainment and the establishment of mentoring relationships. *Journal of Applied Psychology, 81*, 297–308.

Duchscher, J. E., & Cowin, L. S. (2004). The experience of marginalization in new nursing graduates. *Nursing Outlook, 52*, 289–296.

Erkut, S., & Mokros, J. R. (1984). Professors as models and mentors for college students. *American Educational Research Journal, 21*(2), 399–417.

Fassinger, R. E. (1997, August). *Dangerous liaisons: Reflections on feminist mentoring.* Women of the Year Award, address presented at the annual meeting of the American Psychological association, Chicago, IL. Cited in Benishek, L. A., Bieschke, K. J., Park, J., & Slatery, S. M. (2004). A multicultural feminist model of mentoring. *Journal of Multicultural Counseling and Development, 32*, 428–442.

Feldman, D. C. (1976). A contingency theory of socialization. *Administrative Science Quarterly, 21*, 433–452.

Ford, H. R. (2004). Mentoring, diversity, and academic surgery. *Journal of Surgical Research, 118*, 1–8.

Forsyth, A. D., & Stoff, D. M. (2009). Key issues in mentoring in HIV prevention and mental health for new investigators from underrepresented racial/ethnic groups. *American Journal of Public Health, 99*(S1), S87–S91.

Foster, L. (2001). The not-so-invisible professors: White faculty at the Black college. *Urban Education, 36*, 611–629.

Fried, L. P., Francomano, C. A., MacDonald, S. M., Wagner, E. M., Stokes, E. J., Carbone, K. M., et al. (1996). Career development for women in academic medicine: Multiple interventions in a department of medicine. *Journal of the American Medical Association, 276*, 898–905.

Frierson, H. T., Hargrove, B. K., & Lewis, N. R. (1994). Black summer research students' perceptions related to research mentors' race and gender. *Journal of College Student Development, 35*, 475–480.

Fries-Britt, S., & Turner, B. (2002). Uneven stories: Successful Black collegians at a Black and White campus. *Review in Higher Education, 25*, 315–330.

Fullilove, M. T. (1998). Comment abandoning "race" as a variable in public health research: An idea whose time has come. *American Journal of Public Health, 88,* 1297–1298.

Giger, J. N., & Davidhizar, R. (1993). I deserved that promotion. *Minority Nurse Professional, 1,* 26–31.

Girves, J. E., Zepeda, Y., & Gwathmey, J. K. (2005). Mentoring in a post-affirmative action world. *Journal of Social Issues, 61*(3), 449–479.

Greenhaus, J. H., & Parasuraman, S. (1993). Job performance attributions and career advancement prospects: An examination of gender and race effects. *Organizational Behavior and Human Decision Processes, 55,* 273–197.

Grisso, J. A., Hansen, L., Zellinq, I., Bickel, J., & Eisenberg, J. M. (1991). Parental leave policies for faculty in US medical schools. *Annals of Internal Medicine, 114,* 43–45.

Grumbach, K., Coffman, J., Rosenoff, E., & Muñoz, C. (2001). Trends in underrepresented minority participation in health professions schools. In B. D. Smedley, A. Y. Colburn, & C. H. Evans (Eds.), *The right thing to do, the smart thing to do: Enhancing diversity in health professions* (pp. 185–207). Washington, DC: National Academy Press.

Gulam, W., & Zulfiqar, M. (1998). Mentoring—Dr. Plum's elixir and the alchemist's stone. *Mentoring and Tutoring, 5*(3), p. 602. Cited in Cropper, A. (2000). Mentoring as an inclusive device for the excluded: Black students' experience of a mentoring scheme. *Social Work Education, 19*(6), 597–607.

Hamilton, D. L., & Trolier, T. K. (1986). Stereotypes and stereotyping: An overview of the cognitive approach. In J. Dovidio & S. L. Gaertner (Eds.), *Prejudice, discrimination, and racism* (pp. 127–164). New York: Academic Press.

Harshman, E. M., & Rudin, J. P. (2001). Corporate mentoring programs: Legal landmines? *Journal of Employment Discrimination Law, 2*(1), 135–140.

Hayes, D. (2006). *AAMC launches campaign to increase medical school diversity.* Retrieved May 24, 2010, from http://diverseeducation.com/article/6686/

Health Resources and Services Administration. (1995). *Fifth report: Women and medicine* (Publication No. HRSA-P-DM-95-1). Washington, DC: Author.

Heilman, M. E., Block, R. F., Martel, R. F., & Simon, M. C. (1989). Has anything changed? Current characterizations of men, women, and managers. *Journal of Applied Psychology, 74*(6), 935–942.

Heimann, B., & Pittenger, K. (1996). The impact of formal mentorship on socialization and commitment of newcomers. *Journal of Management Issues, 8,* 108–117.

Hellstén, M., & Prescott, A. (2004). Learning at university: The international student experience. *International Education Journal, 5*(3), 344–351.

Herbst, M. (2009, April 26). Immigration: More foreign nurses needed? *Bloomberg Business Week.* Retrieved May 24, 2010, from http://www.businessweek.com/print/bwdaily/dnflash/content/jun2009/db20090619_970033.htm

Hess, F. M., & Leal, D. L. (1997). Minority teachers, minority students, and college matriculation: A new look at the role-modeling hypothesis. *Policy Studies Journal, 25,* 235–248.

Hobbs, F., & Stoops, N. (2002, November). Demographic trends in the 20th century. *Census 2000 special reports.* Washington, DC: United States Census Bureau.

Retrieved May 24, 2010, from http://www.census.gov/prod/2002pubs/censr-4.pdf

Holley, L. C., & Young, D. S. (2005). Career decisions and experiences of social work faculty: A gender comparison. *Journal of Social Work Education, 41*, 297–313.

Hollingsworth, M. A., & Fassinger, R. E. (2002). The role of faculty mentors in the research training of counseling psychology doctoral students. *Journal of Counseling Psychology, 49*(3), 324–330.

Hornblum, A. M. (1998). *Acres of skin: Human experiments at Holmesburg Prison.* New York: Routledge.

Ilgen, D. R., & Youtz, M. A. (1986). Factors affecting the evaluation, and development of minorities in organizations. In K. M. Rowland & G. R. Ferris (Eds.), *Research in personnel and human resources management: A research manual* (Vol. 4, pp. 307–337). Greenwich, CT: JAI Press.

Jenkins, R. (2003). Rethinking ethnicity: Identity, categorization, and power. In J. Stone & R. Dennis (Eds.), *Race and ethnicity: Comparative and theoretical approaches* (pp. 58–71). Malden, MA: Blackwell Publishing.

Jensvold v. Shalala, 829 F. Supp. 131 (D. Md. 1993).

Johnson-Bailey, J., & Cervero, R. M. (2002). Cross-cultural mentoring as a context for learning. *New Directions for Adult and Continuing Education, 96*, 15–26.

Johnson, W. B., & Huwe, J. M. (2002). Toward a typology of mentorship dysfunction in graduate school. *Psychotherapy: Theory/Research/Practice/Training, 39*, 44–55.

Journal of Blacks in Higher Education. (2007). The snail-like progress of Blacks into faculty ranks of higher education. *Journal of Blacks in Higher Education.* Retrieved May 29, 2010, from http://www.jbhe.com/news_views/54_black-faculty-progress.html

Kanter, R. M. (1977). *Men and women of the corporation.* New York: Basic Books.

Koberg, C. S., Boss, R. W., & Goodman, E. (1998). Factors and outcomes associated with mentoring among health-care professionals. *Journal of Vocational Behavior, 53*, 58–72.

Kram, K. E. (1985). *Mentoring at work.* Glenview, IL: Scott, Foresman.

Lang, M. (1986). Black student retention at Black colleges and universities: Problems, issues, and alternatives. *Western Journal of Black Studies, 10*(2), 48–54.

Lark, J. S., & Croteau, J. M. (1998). Lesbian, gay and bisexual doctoral students' mentoring relationships with faculty in counseling psychology: qualitative study. *Counseling Psychologist, 26*(5), 754–776.

Lawler, A. (2005). Diversity: Summer's comments draw attention to gender, racial gaps. *Science, 307*(5709), 492–493.

Lee, W. Y. (1999). Striving toward effective retention: The effect of race on mentoring African American students. *Peabody Journal of Education, 74*, 27–43.

Lenhart, S., & Evans, C. (1991). Sexual harassment and gender discrimination: A primer for women physicians. *Journal of the American Medical Women's Association, 46*, 77–82.

Levinson, W., Kaufman, K., Clark, B., & Tolle, S. W. (1991). Mentors and role models for women in academic medicine. *Western Journal of Medicine, 154*, 423–426.

Lewellen-Williams, C., Johnson, V. A., Deloney, L. A., Thomas, B. R., Goyol, A., & Henry-Tillman, R. (2006). A new model for mentoring underrepresented minority faculty. *Academic Medicine, 81*, 275–279.

Limbert, C. A. (1995). Chrysalis: A peer mentoring group for faculty and staff women. *NWSA [National Women's Studies Association] Journal, 7*(2), 86–99.

Lin, J. J. (2001). *Are all mentors equal? The impact of diversity on mentoring relationships.* Unpublished master's thesis, Rice University, Houston, Texas. Cited in McAllister, C. A., Ahmedani, B. K., Harold, R. D., & Cramer, E. P. (2009). Targeted mentoring: Evaluation of a program. *Journal of Social Work Education, 45*(1), 89–104.

Long, J. S. (1978). Productivity and academic position in the scientific career. *American Sociological Review, 43*(6), 889–908.

Lyons, H. Z., Brenner, B. R., & Fassinger, R. E. (2005). A multicultural test of the theory of work adjustment: Investigating the role of heterosexism and fit perceptions in the job satisfaction of lesbian, gay and bisexual employees. *Journal of Counseling Psychology, 52*, 537–548.

Magrane, D., Lang, J., & Alexander H. (2006). *Women in U.S. academic medicine: Statistics and medical school benchmarking, 2005–2006.* Washington, DC: Association of American Medical Colleges. Retrieved May 24, 2010, from http://www.amc.org/members/gwims/statistics/stats06/start.htm

Malcolm, S., Chubin, D., & Jesse, J. (2004). *Standing our ground: A guidebook for STEM educators in the post-Michigan era.* Washington, DC: American Association for the Advancement of Science.

Margolis, E., & Romero, M. (2001). In the image and likeness: How mentoring functions in the hidden curriculum. In E. Margolis (Ed.), *The hidden curriculum in higher education* (pp. 79–96). New York: Routledge.

Mark, S., Link, H., Morahan, P. S., Pololi, L., Reznik, V., & Tropez-Sims, S. (2001). Innovative mentoring programs to promote gender equity in academic medicine. *Academic Medicine, 76*(1), 39–42.

Mayer, A. P., Blair, J. E., & Files, J. A. (2006). Peer mentoring of women physicians [letter]. *Journal of General Internal Medicine, 21*(9), 1007.

McAllister, C. A., Ahmedani, B. K., Harold, R. D., & Cramer, E. P. (2009). Targeted mentoring: Evaluation of a program. *Journal of Social Work Education, 45*(1), 89–104.

McCroskey, L. L. (1998). *An examination of factors influencing US student perceptions of native and non-native teacher effectiveness.* Paper presented at the annual meeting of the National Communication Association, New York. Cited in Spencer-Rodgers, J., & McGovern, T. (2002). Attitudes toward the culturally different: The role of intercultural communication barriers, affective responses, consensual stereotypes, and perceived threat. *International Journal of Intercultural Relations, 26*, 609–631.

McPhail, B. A. (2004). Setting the record straight: Social work is not a female-dominated position. *Social Work, 49*, 323–326.

Mehri, C. (1997). Could be a model for other companies and other plaintiff classes. *Legal Times*, 530.

Mendenhall, M. E., & Oddon, G. R. (1985). The dimensions of expatriate acculturation. *Academy of Management Review, 10*, 39–47.

Menges, R., & Exum, W. H. (1983). Barriers to the progress of women and minority faculty. *Journal of Higher Education, 54*(2), 123–144.

Mezias, J. M., & Scandura, T. A. (2005). A needs-driven approach to expatriate adjustment and career development: A multiple mentoring perspective. *Journal of International Business Studies, 36*(5), 519–538.

Meznek, J., McGrath, P., & Galaviz, F. (1989). *The puente project*. Sacramento, CA: California Community Colleges, Office of the Chancellor, July (ED 307 920). Presented at Meeting of the Board of Governors of the California Community Colleges, Millbrae, California. Cited in Davidson, M.N. & Foster-Johnson, L. (2001). Mentoring in the preparation of graduate researchers of color. *Review of Educational Research, 71*(4), 549–574.

Miller, N., & Brewer, M. B. (1986). Categorization effects on ingroup and outgroup perception. In J. F. Dovidio & S. L. Gaertner (Eds.), *Prejudice, discrimination, and racism* (pp. 209–229). San Diego, CA: Academic Press.

Morrison, E. W. (1993). Longitudinal study of the effects of information seeking on newcomer socialization. *Journal of Applied Psychology, 78*, 173–183.

Morrow, S. L., Gore, P. A., Jr., & Campbell, B. W. (1996). The application of a socio-cognitive framework to the career development of lesbian women and gay men. *Journal of Vocational Behavior, 48*, 136–148.

Nauta, M. M., Saucier, A. M., & Woodard, L. E. (2001). Interpersonal influences on students' academic and career decisions: The impact of sexual orientation. *Career Development Quarterly, 49*, 352–362.

Nettles, M., & Millett, C. (2002). *Coming up a winner: Student and the Ph.D. gamble.* Ann Arbor, MI: University of Michigan.

Nettles, M., & Millett, C. (2006). *Three magic letters: Getting to Ph.D.* Baltimore, MD: Johns Hopkins University Press.

Ninnes, P., Aitchison, C., & Kalos, S. (1999). Challenges to stereotypes of international students' prior educational experience: Undergraduate education in India. *Higher Education Research & Development, 18*(3), 323–342.

Noe, R. (1988a). Women and mentoring: A review and research agenda. *Academy of Management Review, 13*(1), 65–78.

Noe, R. A. (1988b). An investigation of the determinants of successful assigned mentoring relationships. *Personnel Psychology, 41*, 457–479.

Nonnemaker, L. (2000). Women physicians in academic medicine: New insights from cohort studies. *New England Journal of Medicine, 342*(6), 399–405.

Oberg, K. (1954). *Culture shock (Bobbs-Merrill Reprint Series in the Social Sciences, A-329).* Indianapolis, IN: Bobbs-Merrill. Retrieved March 7, 2009, from https://www.smcm.edu/academics/internationaled/Pdf/cultureshockarticle.pdf

Oberg, K. (1960). Culture shock: Adjustment to new cultural environments. *Practical Anthropology, 7*, 177–182.

O'Connell, A. N., Alpert, J. L., Richardson, M. S., Rotter, N. G., Ruble, D. N., & Under, R. K. (1978). Gender-specific barriers to research in psychology. *Psychological Documents, 8*, 80 (MS. No. 1753). Cited in Rogat, G.A., & Redner, R.L. (1985). How mentoring affects the professional development of women in psychology. *Professional Psychology: Research and Practice, 16*(6), 851–859.

Odom, K., Roberts, L. M., Johnson, R. L., & Cooper, L. A. (2007). Exploring obstacles to opportunities for professional success among ethnic minority medical students. *Academic Medicine, 82*(2), 146–153.

Olson, S., & Fagan, A. P. (2007). *Understanding interventions that encourage minorities to pursue research careers: Summary of a workshop.* Washington, DC: National Academies Press.

Ostroff, C., & Kozlowski, S. (1993). The role of mentoring in the information gathering processes of newcomers during early organizational socialization. *Journal of Vocational Behavior, 42,* 170–183.

Padilla, A. M. (1994). Ethnic minority scholars, research, and mentoring: Current and future issues. *Educational Researcher, 23*(4), 24–27.

Palepu, A., Friedman, R. H., Barnett, R., Carr, P. L., Ash, A. S., Szalacha, L., et al. (1998). Junior faculty members' mentoring relationships and their professional development in US medical schools. *Academic Medicine, 3,* 318–323.

Pololi, L., & Knight, S. (2005). Mentoring faculty in academic medicine: A new paradigm? *Journal of General Internal Medicine, 20*(9), 866–870.

Pololi, L. H., & Knight, S. M., Dennis, K., & Frankel, R. M. (2002). Helping medical school faculty realize their dreams: An innovative, collaborative mentoring program. *Academic Medicine, 77*(5), 377–384.

Preece, X. (1999). *Combating social exclusion in University of Adult Education.* Sussex, UK: University of Sussex. Cited in Cropper, A. (2000). Mentoring as an inclusive device for the excluded: Black students' experience of a mentoring scheme. *Social Work Education, 19*(6), 597–607.

Rabionet, S. E., Santiago, L. E., & Zorrilla, C. D. (2009). A multifaceted mentoring model for minority researchers to address HIV health disparities. *American Journal of Public Health, 99*(S1), S65–S70.

Ragins, B. R. (1997). Diversified mentoring relationships in organizations: A peer perspective. *Academy of Management Review, 22,* 482–521.

Ragins, B. R., & Cotton, J. L. (1991). Easier said than done: Gender differences in perceived barriers to gaining a mentor. *Academy of Management Journal, 34*(4), 939–951.

Ragins, B. R., & McFarlin, D. B. (1990). Perceptions of mentor roles in cross-gender mentoring relationships. *Journal of Vocational Behavior, 37,* 321–339.

Richardson, A. (1974). *British immigrants and Australia: A psycho-social inquiry.* Canberra, ACT: Australian National University Press.

Rivera-Goba, M. V., & Nieto, S. (2007). Mentoring Latina nurses: A multicultural perspective. *Journal of Latinos and Education, 6*(1), 35–53.

Robinson, L. H. (1973). Institutional variation in the status of academic women. In A. Rossi & A. Calderwood (Eds.), *Academic women on the move* (pp. 199–238). New York: Russell Sage Foundation.

Rogat, G.A., & Redner, R.L. (1985). How mentoring affects the professional development of women in psychology. *Professional Psychology: Research and Practice, 16*(6), 851–859.

Rowe, M. (1990). Barriers to equality: The power of subtle discrimination to maintain unequal opportunity. *Employee Responsibilities and Rights Journal, 3,* 153–163.

Rubin, D. L., & Smith, K. A. (1990). Effects of accent, ethnicity, and lecture type on undergraduates' perceptions of nonnative English-speaking teaching assistants. *International Journal of Intercultural Relations, 14,* 337–353.

Russell, J. E. A. (1994). Career counseling for women in management. In W. B. Walsh & S. H. Osipow (Eds.), *Career counseling for women* (pp. 263–326). Hillsdale, NJ: Lawrence Erlbaum Associates.

Russo, N. F., Olmedo, E. L., Stapp, J., & Fulcher, R. (1981). Women and minorities in psychology. *American Psychologist, 36,* 1315–1363.

Ryan, J. (2000). Assessment. In J. Ryan (Ed.), *A guide to teaching international students*. Oxford, UK: Oxford Centre for Staff and Learning Development University.

Salsberg, E., & Grover, A. (2006). Physician workforce shortages: Implications and issues for academic health centers and policy makers. *Academic Medicine, 81,* 782–787.

Scandura, T. A., & Ragins, B. R. (1993). The effects of sex and gender role orientation on mentorship in male-dominated occupations. *Journal of Vocational Behavior, 43,* 251–265.

Schein, E. H. (1971). The individual, the organization, and the career: A conceptual scheme. *Journal of Applied Behavioral Science, 7,* 401–426.

Sedlacek, W. E. (1999). Black students on White campuses: 20 years of research. *Journal of College Student Development, 40,* 538–550.

Shafer, M. (2004, March 9). Havasupai blood samples misused. *Indian Country Today*. Retrieved May 24, 2010, from http://www.indiancountrytoday.com/archive/28177554.html

Shavers, V. L., Fagan, P., Lawrence, D., McCaskill-Stevens, W., McDonald, P., Browne, D., et al. (2005). Barriers to racial/ethnic minority application and competition for NIH research funding. *Journal of the National Medical Association, 97,* 1063–1077.

Simon, C. E., Roff, L. L., & Perry, A. R. (2008). Psychosocial and career mentoring: Female African American social work education administrators' experiences. *Journal of Social Work Education, 44*(1), 9–22.

Smedley, B. D., Stith, A. Y., & Nelson, A. R. (Eds.). (2003). *Unequal treatment: Confronting racial and ethnic disparities in health care*. Washington, DC: National Academies Press.

Solomon, L. C. (1976). *Male and female graduate students: The question of equal opportunity*. New York: Praeger.

Solomon, L. C. (1978). Attracting women to psychology: Effects of university behavior and the labor market. *American Psychologist, 33,* 990–999.

Sosik, J. J., & Godshalk, V. M. (2000). The role of gender in mentoring: Implications for diversified and homogenous mentoring relationships. *Journal of Vocational Behavior, 57,* 102–122.

Spencer-Rodgers, J. (2001). Consensual and individual stereotypic beliefs about international students among American host nations. *International Journal of Intercultural Relations, 25,* 639–657.

Spencer-Rodgers, J., & McGovern, T. (2002). Attitudes toward the culturally different: The role of intercultural communication barriers, affective responses, consensual stereotypes, and perceived threat. *International Journal of Intercultural Relations, 26,* 609–631.

Steinpreis, R. E., Anders, K. A., & Ritzke, D. (1999). The impact of gender on the review of curricula vitae of job applicants and tenure candidates: A national empirical study. *Sex Roles, 41*(7/8), 509–528.

Stoff, D. M., Forsyth, A., Marquez, E. D., & McClure, S. (2009). Introduction: The case for diversity in research on mental health and HIV/AIDS. *American Journal of Public Health, 99*(S1), S8–S15.

Stolley, P. D. (1999). Race in epidemiology. *International Journal of Health Services, 29,* 905–909.

Sue, D. W., Capodilupo, C. M., Torino, G. C., Bucceri, J. M., Holder, A. M., Nadal, K. L., et al. (2007). Racial microaggressions in everyday life: Implications for clinical practice. *American Psychologist, 62,* 271–286.

Syverson, P. D. (1982). Two decades of doctorates in psychology: A comparison with national trends. *American Psychologist, 37,* 1203–1212.

Tajfel, H., & Turner, J. C. (1986). The social identity theory of intergroup behavior. In S. Worchel & W. G. Austin (Eds.), *Psychology of group relations* (pp. 7–24). Chicago, IL: Nelson-Hall.

Terrell, M. C., & Hassell, T. R. (1994). Mentoring undergraduate minority students: An overview, survey, and model program. In M. A. Wunsch (Ed.), *Mentoring revisited: Making an impact on individuals and institutions.* San Francisco, CA: Jossey-Bass.

Thomas, D. A. (1990). The impact of race on managers' experiences of developmental relationships (mentoring and sponsorship): An intra-organizational study. *Journal of Organizational Behavior, 11*(6), 479–492.

Thomas, D. A. (1993). Racial dynamics in cross-race developmental relationships. *Administrative Science Quarterly, 38*(2), 169–194.

Thomas, S. B. & Quinn, S. C. (1991). The Tuskegee Syphilis Study, 1932 to 1972: Implications for HIV education and AIDS risk education programs in the black community. *American Journal of Public Health, 81*(11), 1498–1504.

Tillman, L. C. (2001). Mentoring African American faculty in predominantly white institutions. *Research in Higher Education, 42,* 295–325.

Tonkovich, J., & Slater, R. (2004, November). *Gender communication differences: Why we need more speech-language pathologists.* Poster presentation at the 2004 American Speech-Language-Hearing Association meeting. November, Philadelphia. Cited in Wright-Harp, W., & Cole, P.A. (2008). A mentoring model for enhancing success in graduate education. *Contemporary Issues in Communication Science and Disorders, 35,* 4–16.

Treadwell, H. M., Braithwaite, R. L., Braithwaite, K., Oliver, D., & Holliday, R. (2009). Leadership development for health researchers at historically Black colleges and universities. *American Journal of Public Health, 99*(S1), S53–S57.

United States Department of Education. (2010). *White House initiative on historically black colleges and universities.* Retrieved May 24, 2010, from http://ed.gov/about/ inits/list/whhbcu/edlite-exec-order.html

United States Department of Health and Human Services, Health Resources and Services Administration. (2006). *The registered nurse population: Findings from the 2004 National Survey of Registered Nurses (NSSRN).* Washington, DC: Bureau of Health Professions, Division of Nursing. Retrieved July 9, 2010, from http://bhpr.hrsa.gov/healthworkforce/rnsurvey04/

Van Maanen, J., & Schein, E. H. (1979). Toward a theory of organizational socialization. In B. M. Staw (Ed.), *Research in organizational behavior* (Vol. 1, pp. 209–264). Greenwich, CT: JAI Press.

Viator, R. F., & Scandura, T. A. (1991). A study of mentor-protégé relationships in large public accounting firms. *Accounting Horizons, 5*(3), 20–30.

Villarruel, A. M., Canales, M., & Torres, S. (2001). Bridges and barriers: Educational mobility of Hispanic nurses. *Journal of Nursing Education, 40*(6), 245–251.

Wainer, J. (2004). Work of female rural doctors. *Australian Journal of Rural Health, 12*, 49–53.

Wallace, D., Abel, R., & Ropers-Huilman, B. (2000). Clearing a path for success: Deconstructing borders through undergraduate mentoring. *Review of Higher Education, 24*, 87–102.

Wallace, J. E. (2001). The benefits of mentoring for female lawyers. *Journal of Vocational Behavior, 58*, 366–391.

Walters, K. L., & Simoni, J. M. (2009). Decolonizing strategies for mentoring American Indians and Alaska Natives in HIV and mental health research. *American Journal of Public Health, 99*(S1), S71–S76.

Wan, T., Chapman, D. W., & Biggs, D. A. (1992). Academic stress of international students attending US universities. *Research in Higher Education, 33*, 607–623.

Ward, G. G. (1936). Marion Sims and the origin of modern gynecology. *Bulletin of the New York Academy of Medicine, 12*(3), 93–104.

Wright-Harp, W., & Cole, P. A. (2008). A mentoring model for enhancing success in graduate education. *Contemporary Issues in Communication Science and Disorders, 35*, 4–16.

Wyatt, G. E., Williams, J. K., Henderson, T., & Sumner, L. (2009). On the outside looking in: Promoting HIV/AIDS research initiated by African American investigators. *American Journal of Public Health, 99*(S1), S48–S53.

Zachary, L. J. (2000). *The mentor's guide: Facilitating effective learning relationships.* San Francisco: Jossey-Bass Publishers.

FOUR

Case Study Four

An International Mentee's Experience

Beatrice Gabriela Ioan

This case study focuses on the writer's experience as both a Romanian trainee in a U.S.-based master's degree program in bioethics and, subsequently, her experience as a Romanian mentor to others in Romania. This experience required that she integrate her U.S. education and then adapt it to the Romanian cultural and educational contexts.

The case study first provides an overview of the Romanian context as it existed at the start of this author's studies. It then focuses on the nature of her experience as a mentee and her later efforts to adapt what she had learned to the Romanian context upon her reentry to her country. The case study concludes with a summary of the progress made to date in the development of bioethics in the Romanian context.

THE ROMANIAN SOCIOPOLITICAL FRAMEWORK
BEFORE AND AFTER 1989

In the communist countries dominated by the former USSR, the emphasis was placed on guarantees of positive rights, such as the right to education, to medical care, to a living wage, and to benefit from paid holidays. However, the state retained the right to intervene in individuals' lives, which led to the infringement of the negative (natural) human rights such as the right to liberty.

The communist regime in Romania was established in 1945. This regime promised the well-being of all the members of society but this promise proved to be illusory; political repression of various aspects of life, ranging from the most subtle to the most obvious, became the rule in the society. This regime lasted for 44 years, till 1989, but the long-term effects of the changes at all the levels of economic and social life that occurred during communism can be felt even today, after 20 years from its fall.

During the communist era, the fields of medical ethics and bioethics were deeply affected. These disciplines were considered insignificant because the supreme goal of the Communist Party was to establish a socialist society in which the individual him/her was unimportant. To understand the difficulties faced in attempts to reintroduce bioethics in Romania and the need for major changes in attitudes toward this field, it is important to point out some of the problems that permeated the Romanian health care system, Romanian society as a whole and, implicitly, the social and medical ethics and morals during communism.

During the communist regime some of the Romanian legislative regulations incorporated the values and moral principles of bioethics but these never had a significant influence in practice and remained almost unknown, while glaring infringements of human rights occurred. Actually, when analyzing the Romanian legislation during the communist regime, one can observe an obvious inconsistency in regulations related to life and health of individuals. In certain situations the law sustained the ethical principles recognized today, while in others the infringement of human rights was favored by law, according to necessities of the socialist society.

As an example of this inherent contradiction, although Law 3/1978 required informed consent from patients for medical procedures, Romanian medicine remained highly paternalistic; health care professionals rarely integrated the requirement of informed consent into their practice. As a result, recognition of a patient's right to autonomy remains difficult even now. Although the law required a patient's informed consent prior to the performance of any diagnostic or therapeutic intervention, it also obliged women of childbearing age to submit to medical examinations and adhere to the pro-birth policies of the Communist Party. One of the most obvious infringements of human rights occurred as the result of decree 779, which was issued in 1967. This decree strictly forbade abortion, essentially nullifying women's procreative liberty.[1] The decree was launched when the decrease in Romania's birth rate reached an alarmingly low level; this

---

[1] The rate of abortion peaked in 1965, when there were approximately four abortions per every newborn child. Prior to 1967, abortion was the most popular method of birth control in Romania (Ghebrea, 2000). However, decree 779 permitted abortion in only two circumstances: when the pregnancy endangered the life of the woman and when the woman already had at least four children. The law reflected the pro-birth policy of the Romanian Communist Party and its view of the fetus as socialist property belonging to the state. However, the decree did not bring about the anticipated results. Although a sharp decrease in the rate of abortion occurred in 1967, falling to 0.4 abortions per each birth, the rate subsequently rose yet again in 1969 to one abortion per one birth. Attempts to enforce the decree through prohibitions against the use of birth control methods and abortion, mandated medical examinations of women and the imposition of quotas on physicians for the delivery of newborns ultimately led to the deaths of many women due to illegal abortion and a high rate of infant mortality (Ioan & Astărăstoae, 2006).

situation was deemed to be unacceptable by the socialist society which needed new members and wished to be a positive example for its neighboring communist countries.

Another area that was affected heavily by Communist ideology was psychiatry. At the time, it was often used as a political weapon, resulting in the creation of a "political psychiatry." This was fueled by three tenets of the communist society: the individual had no rights, the Communist Party decided the fate of people, and science (in this case psychiatry) was compelled to follow the socialist ideology. The "cult of masses" led to the emergence of new and absurd principles, such as the adherence of all individuals to socialism, the superiority of socialism, and the inevitable evolution of any society to socialism.

Psychiatric ethics was forced to comply with these new principles, this new morality. As a consequence, politically or religiously motivated opposition came to be classified as psychopathological manifestations, normality being represented by conformists, that is, those who adhered to the requirements of the communist system. Individuals who voiced opposition to the communist regime were labeled as paranoid (Cucu & Dănilă, 2009). Law 3/1978 permitted the sequestration of the individual in an emergency; "medical emergency" was recharacterized as "political emergency." Decree No. 12/1965 provided for the involuntary admission to the hospital of an individual who was deemed to be "dangerous," a charge that could be made by any family member or neighbor and against which the individual implicated had no right to defend. Decree 313/1980 permitted a sole psychiatrist to mandate the individual's treatment, which in some cases occurred at the behest of the governmental security forces, the infamous Securitate. Not surprisingly, medical repression used by the communist regime to achieve its goals led to violations of medical ethics, and thus discredited the medical profession. Abuses included the involuntary and unwarranted hospitalization of individuals and the administration of neuroleptic medication or electric shock without medical justification (Cucu & Dănilă, 2009).

Health care facilities in East European countries during communism were seen and organized as genuine "health factories" in which professionals' work was evaluated based on the number of beds, the number of patients treated, and the degree of endowment of hospitals. Important issues such as age, sex, personal characteristics of patients, or ethical dilemmas that inevitably arose during the provision of medical care were neglected. This purely bureaucratic approach of the health care system, which still persists in the former communist countries (Borovecki, ten Have, & Oreskovic, 2005) contributed significantly to the neglect of medical ethics and bioethics in the Romanian health care system.

Communist health care policies focused to a large degree on children, women, and workers, without attention to the needs of all members of society. In these circumstances, doctors who were serving the working class were forced to work in unsanitary conditions, with an exhausting work schedule; as a result, the quality of medical care was frequently poor, and frequent violations of ethical principles occurred. As an example, some patients were unintentionally infected with hepatitis B, hepatitis C, and/or HIV due to poor sterilization of medical equipment. The communist medical education played an important role in maintaining this state of affairs due to the emphasis placed on ideology rather than on principles of medical ethics (Horber & Zilahi, 2007).

In 1989, Romania shifted from communism to democracy. It was first a political change, followed by a difficult transition period in all sectors of society. Romania and Romanian society opened to the rest of the world and step-by-step the need to adopt universal principles of democracy became obvious. During the transition, since 1989, many of the social aspects established during communism have disappeared gradually (Ioan & Astărăstoae, 2006).

Bioethics is one of the fields that followed an ascendant evolution after 1989. Initially, this was attributable to Romania's political interest in joining the European Union and the associated requirements of the European Union and other international bodies. As a consequence, the principles of bioethics have been stated first in legislation; their operationalization and implementation was held in abeyance for a while, primarily due to the lack of professionals and training programs in this field. The next step, still unfinished, was the involvement of specialists in the dissemination of bioethics and the creation of bodies to promote it, such as clinical ethics committees, research ethics committees, bioethics committee of the Romanian College of Physicians, and the bioethics committee of the Ministry of Health. Along with these, the introduction of the study of bioethics into the university curriculum sought to familiarize the future physicians with theoretical issues in bioethics and their practical application in order to enable them to recognize and solve the ethical problems in their future daily practice (Ioan & Astărăstoae, 2008).

THE AMERICAN EXPERIENCE OF A ROMANIAN PHYSICIAN-TRAINEE

In 2001, a collaboration between the Department of Bioethics of Case Western Reserve University (CWRU) of Cleveland, Ohio, USA and the College of Physicians (Colegiul Medicilor) of Iaşi, Romania was established to train Romanian professionals in the master's degree program in bioethics through CWRU. At the end of the academic training period, the graduates were to return to Romania to build a network of professionals in the field of bioethics. The focus of this project is that of mentorship, designed to disseminate bioethics education and to build a critical mass of individuals trained in research ethics in the countries where this field is absent or poorly developed. To that end, the U.S. faculty members served as mentors to the new specialists in bioethics, who become, in turn, mentors for students and professionals in their countries of origin.

My training period (2003–2004) in bioethics in the United States was not an easy one but it was, for sure, of great benefit to my professional development. This is because I had the chance to learn bioethics and the American perspective in this field from highly experienced professionals with various backgrounds, including philosophy, medicine, sociology, psychology, and epidemiology, who were willing to share both their knowledge and experience to others. This approach gave me the opportunity to explore this field in a multidisciplinary fashion and to understand that contrary to the then-prevalent view in Romania, bioethics does not belong to medicine alone, but rather to all life sciences.

Although I taught bioethics in medical school, I had had no formal education in this field but learned it by myself. The MA program in bioethics trained me to become a professional in bioethics and, maybe more importantly, to share the knowledge that I gained with others. Although it is not the purpose of this paper to detail the content of the MA program, I should mention that it was a complex program, which resulted in a fundamental change in my understanding about ethics and bioethics. It would be significant to mention that above all theoretical and practical knowledge, I learned that working in this field and teaching bioethics has to be based on pillars, such as inter-disciplinarity, complexity, an open mind to all possibilities and aspects of a problem, tolerance for different views, and mutual respect.

ADAPTING THE U.S. EXPERIENCE TO THE ROMANIAN CONTEXT

As I already mentioned, after 1 year of training I came back home planning to become a mentor and real "change agent" in bioethics. The greatest challenge in this endeavor was to facilitate an understanding in Romania that the knowledge gained in the United States was relevant to the Romanian context, that is, to convince others that bioethics is a reality of our world, that the situations and ethical dilemmas in other countries can also arise in Romania, and that the principles of bioethics are necessary and appropriate for the Romanian medical and scientific environment. This was particularly critical, although an optional course in bioethics had been available as part of the medical curriculum in Iasi since 1990, bioethics became a compulsory subject of study for medical school students only in 2004 and is gradually being added to the curriculum for students in the fields of dentistry, pharmacy, medical bioengineering, nursing, and midwifery (Ioan & Astărăstoae, 2008).

It became evident, therefore, that the knowledge achieved in the U.S. program had to be adapted to Romanian reality, so that bioethics would not remain at the theoretical level only, but would be used as a tool to resolve practical dilemmas. This required nothing less than the development of a "Romanian Bioethics," anchored in the realities of Romanian society and responding to its requirements.

The first step in this approach was to identify the specifics of the Romanian society that are relevant to the field of bioethics. The most important components include religion, socioeconomic features, characteristics of the Romanian family, and the paternalistic tradition of Romania's medical practice.

Religious Affiliation of Romanians

According to the 2002 census, 86.7% of the Romanians declared themselves as belonging to the Orthodox Christian religion (http://www .recensamant.ro/datepr/tbl6.html). In the past decade, in particular, there has been a resurgence of religiosity (Voicu, 2007). Accordingly, the recognition and discussion of the principles of Christian Orthodoxy become essential in various matters relating to human and animal life. For this reason, the field of bioethics considers the principles and opinions of the Bioethics Commission of the Romanian Orthodox Church (available at http://www.patriarhia.ro). Formerly, Romanian Orthodox Church's involvement in politics was limited and the Church's engagement was restricted to social and moral debate. In recent years, however, the Bioethics Commission of the Romanian Orthodox Church has developed views on issues of great interest, such as euthanasia, abortion, and organ transplantation; its perspective now serves as a reference point in addressing these issues in Romania.

Socioeconomic Features

After the fall of the communist regime in 1989, Romania entered a period of transition to democracy and a market economy. This has produced profound changes in the economic, social, and family life. Frustrations about living conditions and food shortages that accumulated during the communist regime continued to some extent during the transition (Simion, 2004). An unstable economic environment has also developed, which has led to job instability and an increased number of people without health insurance.

The low level of financing for the health sector and the poor equipment of hospitals have created ethical issues of particular importance in the allocation of material resources. As the result of poor and deteriorating working conditions and wages, an increase in the migration of Romanian medical personnel to West European countries has occurred in recent years, leading to a further decrease in human resources within the Romanian health care system. At present, Romania ranks 31st among the 33 European countries, with a density of 1.9 doctors for every 1,000 inhabitants; only Albania and Bosnia-Herţegovina register lower values than Romania (Resursele Umane pentru Sănătate, 2004). More than 4% of all board-certified medical doctors, that is, more than 1,000 doctors have already left Romania. In more than one-third of Romania's counties, there are no physicians in medical subspecialities at all (Dragomirişteanu, Fărcăşanu & Galan, 2008).

The Characteristics of the Typical Romanian Family

In Romania the traditional family model is characterized by strong affectionate and economical relationships between parents and children (Ioan & Astărăstoae, 2006). In many cases, children remain near their parents, even after they have reached the age of majority. Attachment to family is also demonstrated by several objective data, such as an increased tendency to marry, a low proportion of permanent celibacy, young age at marriage, a low divorce rate compared to other European countries, a low proportion of cohabiting relationships, and a relatively small number of children born outside marriage (Ghebrea, 2000).

As a result, family involvement in the care of the patient is very important. The motivation for the frequent involvement of family medical care of patients is, on the one hand, close relations between family members and the patient's desire to be morally sustained by family and, secondly, the paternalistic tradition of medicine that has been inherited from the communist regime.

Romania's Paternalistic Tradition of Medicine

The long period of paternalism that characterized Romanian medical practice is a serious constraint to the introduction of principles which evaluate the patient–doctor relationship on ethical grounds and considers the patient to be the physician's partner in the therapeutic decision-making process. During the Communist era, Romanian medicine suffered from a deficit of communication between doctor and patient. For example, information regarding a diagnosis was often withheld from the patient and revealed only to his or her family members; frequently, oncology patients died without understanding the nature of their illness or the reason for their impending death. Medical students were trained exclusively for the technical aspects of their profession, without taking into account many other psychological, social, and religious aspects, all of which may be crucial for the evolution of a clinical case. Resistance to reform the doctor–patient relationship so as to integrate well-accepted principles of bioethics comes especially from professionals who worked for a long period of time during the communist regime, when the patient had to listen and comply with what the doctor prescribed without consideration of the patient's wishes.

INTRODUCING BIOETHICS INTO ROMANIAN MEDICAL PRACTICE

The Impetus for Change

As indicated, issues related to medical ethics and bioethics have been for a long period of time neglected and unrecognized in Romanian medical practice. Therefore, the creation of an ethical foundation for medical practice and research requires identification of the most suitable method of providing information that will lead to real change in professionals' attitudes and behavior. In order to achieve beneficial results, educational intervention should begin as early as faculty studies, but must also focus on professionals already working in medical facilities. The need for a change of perspective in medical and life sciences and for placing them on real ethical grounds came from two directions: society and law.

The importance of changing the mentality of medical professionals is reflected in the large number of cases analyzed by the Superior Disciplinary Commission of the Romanian College of Physicians [Colegiul Medicilor din România]. This Commission is responsible for the analysis of cases involving patients' complaints against their physicians due to a breach of their rights and the ethical, moral, and deontological principles of medicine. In most cases analyzed by the Superior Disciplinary Commission,[2] patients complain about the infringement of their right to be informed, the provision to the patient of incomplete information, infringement of the patient's right to informed consent before the performance of any diagnostic or therapeutic act, and violations of medical data privacy. Such cases and the growing number of patients' complaints, increasing from 112 in 2006 to 135 in 2007, to 171 in 2008, serve as strong evidence that, in the Romanian health care system, there is at the present time a real need for health care professionals to know and to respect the principles of bioethics, imposed at least in part by the pressure of patients and society as a whole.

---

[2]Details relating to the composition and procedures of the Superior Disciplinary Commission can be found at http://www.cmr.ro

Before and after joining the European Union, Romania was required to align its legislation with European legal standards, particularly those relating to human rights. Some of these legal regulations which represent progress in the field are listed below.

The Law 17/2001, through which Romania ratified the Oviedo Convention on Human Rights and Biomedicine, requires that all legislation with reference to health and human life be subject, in the planning phase, to evaluation by an ethics committee.

According to the Law No. 46/2003 on patient's rights, the physician must inform the patient about his health status and consult her/him on the therapeutic intervention to be used. The patient has the right to confidentiality of personal data even with respect to members of his or her family if the patient does not wish otherwise. This law also contains provisions relating to the physician's and patient's relationship with the media, the patient's participation in medical education, and the patient's right to private life and procreative liberty. To cope with dilemmas of medical practice, the law provides for the establishment of hospital clinical ethics committees.

Law No. 206/2004, on good conduct in scientific research, technological development, and innovation, provides the ethical standards in biomedical research. These are in line with the internationally recognized and accepted standards and guidelines and require that research projects be approved by a local research ethics committee or the national research ethics committee, depending upon the type and complexity of the research project.

Law No. 95/2006 on health care reform enunciates the ethical guidelines to be followed in human organ, tissue, and cell transplantation, including the necessity for setting up the Commission for approval of donation of organs from living donors, one of its members being a physician trained in bioethics. This law also contains provisions on malpractice and deontological responsibility of medical personnel (www.cdep.ro).

As indicated above, Romanian law currently mandates, on the one hand, that health care professionals respect bioethics principles in medical practice and biomedical research. On the other hand, Romanian law requires that health care professionals be trained in bioethics both in current medical practice and in research project evaluation. In this way, Romanian legislation provides a strong motivation for training specialists in bioethics.

Following the identification of the need for a change, the most appropriate methods to achieve it must be identified. Without claiming to identify all interventional methods, the following approaches are useful in our efforts to disseminate information on bioethics in the Romanian medical field and society.

Educational Approaches

Moving From a Top-Down to a Bottom-Up Approach

In order to transform medical practice based on a change in professionals' beliefs. The bottom-up approach is totally contrary to the communist top-down approach, where moral principles were not the result of an inner transformation of individuals in contact with society but a requirement that the individual change to meet the Marxist/Communist ideology. This approach has failed in all former communist countries.

The history of communist regimes demonstrates that change in ideas, beliefs, and attitudes cannot be mandated. This is the reason why we considered that dissemination and implementation of bioethics in Romanian medical practice and research should be started from internalization of moral and ethical principles by professionals. In this way, the change in the health care system would come from its professionals and, as such, stand a better chance to endure over time.

Using Particular Teaching Methods

This includes a case-based approach and interactive teaching, which enable the students to understand and integrate the information taught during the course. The most useful approach to date incorporates concrete examples and cases to demonstrate the practical utility of theoretical knowledge and to anchor the theory in everyday practice. Since this is a particular method of teaching, centered on the practical examples and case analysis, it was necessary from the outset to set guidelines for the discussions: respect for the ideas contrary to their own, and an opportunity for all participants in the discussion to express their views and be heard.

To convince practitioners and researchers that bioethics is not a Western invention that is being forced on Romanian medical practice, it has been necessary to move from exclusive reliance on known cases of Western literature to cases of Romanian practice. This requires problem solving in the context of the Romanian social, economic, and religious environment. In this way, it is shown that difficult moral dilemmas could arise in the context of Romania's medical practice and that the attitudes of Romanian health care professionals must change so that human life is more highly valued and the patient is perceived as the physician's partner in providing health care.

This approach helps students to develop an awareness of the shortcomings of the health system and to recognize that everyday medical practice in Romania is far behind current laws and ethical principles related to health care. They have begun to identify both the ethical problems that may arise during their clinical rotations and possible solutions, using the knowledge that they have gained during bioethics courses and seminars.

Additionally, continuing education lectures that were often required by professional associations in various medical specialties now include a component focusing on principles of bioethics and have as lecturers faculty specialists in bioethics. The bioethics courses for both students and professionals include material relating to health legislation.

FOLLOWING THE EXAMPLE OF MENTORS

The first—and only—master's degree program in bioethics in Romania was launched at the University of Medicine and Pharmacy in Iasi during academic year 2005–2006. The goal of this program was the development of cadre specialists in bioethics who could serve on clinical ethics committees, research ethics committees, or teach and conduct bioethics research in an academic setting.

The program recruits students from a wide range of disciplines. The implementation of this approach has been hampered by the widespread belief that bioethics belongs to medicine and, therefore, that only doctors can participate in a master's program in bioethics. This false belief most likely originates from confusion between medical ethics and bioethics. Because the master's degree program in bioethics was organized in the Medical School in Iasi, the majority of the students were graduates in medical studies. However, the program has also accepted and trained professionals from psychology, theology, and engineering. This multidisciplinarity has facilitated the exchange of diverse views and ideas and the identification of issues, which go far beyond the boundaries of medicine.

Generally speaking, the structure of the curriculum of Romania's Master's in Bioethics Program mirrors the curriculum of the bioethics program of CWRU. However, it also includes a number of particular issues characteristic to the Romanian society, as discussed previously. In view of the interdisciplinarity of the field, the faculty includes professors with diverse disciplinary backgrounds, including medicine, psychology, philosophy, sociology, law, and theology, with all sharing the concerns for the field of ethics and bioethics.

In 2007, bioethics was introduced as a compulsory 2-week module in the residency curricula of all medical specialties. In 2008, an optional course on communication in the medical field was made available to medical students. The course is taught by a multidisciplinary team consisting of a bioethicist, a specialist in therapeutic education, a sociologist, a psychologist, and a theologian. During this course, the students learn various aspects and issues in communication with a particular emphasis on communication in the medical field.

Since 2003, we have published in Iasi the *Romanian Journal of Bioethics* [*Revista Română de Bioetică*],[3] the first publication in this field in our country.

---

[3] The electronic version of the journal can be found at http://www.bioetica.ro

The first issue of the journal was published in March 2003. Since that time, the journal has been published every trimester, having as its main goal the dissemination of bioethical information to professionals within the health care system and to the public at large.

CONCLUSION

Successful mentorship requires education through appropriate methods and the creation of successive waves of new mentors. The development of a critical mass of specialists in bioethics, initiated in 2001 through the establishment of a successful Romanian–American cooperation, can be sustained by those students who return home from their U.S. training, equipped with both the skills and eagerness to play a key role in the bold development of this new discipline and the insight necessary to dispel the old and false beliefs. At the time of this writing, 10 professionals have graduated with a master's degree in bioethics through this international collaboration, forming a cadre of skilled professionals prepared to address ethical dilemmas arising in the Romanian context and to move the field of Romanian bioethics forward. Our efforts have been fruitful because we have anchored theory to the realities of Romanian society and adapted knowledge and theory to everyday practice. Starting from what is universally valid and recognized, we have started to build what is true and valid in Romania, according to local social, economic, and religious realities. While neither embracing nor opposing globalization, we recognize that the integration of universal principles is necessary and useful to the extent that national identity is preserved. This approach will enhance the likelihood that bioethics is accepted as a legitimate discipline and that the program will continue to prove successful.

REFERENCES

Borovecki, A., ten Have, H., & Oreskovic, S. (2005). Ethics and the structures of health care in the European countries in transition: Hospital ethics committees in Croatia. *British Medical Journal, 331,* 227–229.

Cucu, I. C., & Dănilă, M. (2009) *Istoria tragică a psihiatriei româneşti în perioada comunismului* [The tragic history of Romanian psychiatry during the communist regime]. Retrieved December 9, 2009, from http://www.psihologie.net

Dragomirişteanu, A., Fărcăşanu, D. O., & Galan A. (2008). *Migraţia medicilor din România* [Migration among Romanian physicians]. Retrieved from www.cmr.ro

Ghebrea, G. (2000). *Regim social-politic şi viaţă privată.* [The social-political regime and private life]. Bucharest, Romania: Editura Universităţii din Bucureşti.

Horber, O., & Zilahi, K. (2007). *Sensibilitatea socială în istoria medicinei secolelor XIX–XX: Ideologie politică sau umanism european? Etica medicală între constrângere şi convingere* [The social sensitivity in the history of medicine of the 19th–20th centuries: Political ideology or European humanism? Medical ethics between coercion and conviction]. *Revista Română de Bioetică, 5*(2), 13–17.

Ioan, B., & Astărăstoae, V. (2006). *Procreative liberty in Romania: Between abortion and medically assisted human reproduction.* Retrieved November 8, 2010, from https://www.medecine.univ-paris5.fr/IMG/pdf/text_procreative_liberty_in_romania_between_abortion_and_medically_assisted_reproduction.pdf

Ioan, B., & Astărăstoae, V. (2008). *Esperienze didattiche a confronto: le Universita Romene, în L'educazione alla bioetica in Europa* (pp. 93–103). red. Paolo Girolami. SEEd SRL, Torino, Italy.

Law no 3 of July 6, 1978 on ensuring the population's health, published in Official Bulletin no 54 of July 10, 1978, www.cdep.ro

Law no 17/2001 on ratification of Oviedo Convention on Human Rights and Biomedicine, www.cdep.ro

Law no 46/2003 on patient's rights, www.cdep.ro

Law no 206/2004 on good conduct in scientific research, technological development and innovation, www.cdep.ro

Law 95/2006 on healthcare reform, www.cdep.ro

Populaţia după religie la Recensământul din 2002. Retrieved December 28, 2009, from http://www.recensamant.ro/datepr/tbl6.html

Simion, M. (2004). *Profilul demografic al României* [Demographic profile of Romania]. Retrieved January 6, 2009, from http://www.iccv.ro/oldiccv/romana/revista/rcalvit/pdf/cv2004.1-2.a03.pdf

Voicu, M. (2007). *România religioasă* [Religious Romania]. Iaşi, România: Editura Institutul European.

FIVE

Developing a Mentoring Program, Training, and Evaluating Mentors, Mentees, and Mentoring Relationships

The development and evaluation of a mentoring program requires that attention be focused on multiple levels: the institution or organization that houses the mentoring program, the program through which the mentoring occurs or is organized, the mentor, the mentee, and the mentor–mentee relationship.

PROGRAM DEVELOPMENT

Organizational Considerations

It has been suggested that the sponsoring institution of a mentoring program is not only critical to its success, but also that the traditional dyadic model of mentoring should be reconceptualized into a triadic model comprised of the sponsoring institution, the mentor, and the mentee (Walker, Kelly, & Hume, 2002). Accordingly, consideration must be given to various organization/institution-level variables in developing a mentoring program. These include the extent to which structural segregation exists, the nature of the management system, and the organizational culture.

Structural segregation "refers to the achievement of proportional heterogeneity in employment positions across rank, department, and specialization" (Ragins, 1997, pp. 93–94; see also Cox, 1991, 1993). Structurally segregated organizations relegate, whether inadvertently or by design, minority individuals to lower ranks than their majority counterparts and erect "glass ceilings" that hinder their ability to gain access to higher-ranking positions and to "fast-track" on their career trajectory (Ragins & Sundstrom, 1989). Structural segregation may impact the composition of mentoring relationships by limiting the minority individuals' numbers who can achieve higher ranks and, consequently, who may be available to mentor minority students or professionals (Ragins, 1997).

Management systems may be mechanistic or may reflect a "new paradigm" (Ragins, 1997). Mechanistic organizations are hierarchical; power is centralized and communication proceeds strictly along vertical lines of authority (Burns & Stalker, 1961). In contrast, the control in organizations with "new paradigm" management systems is decentralized; communication may occur laterally across department lines, and frequently consists of advice and information, rather than instructions and decisions (Bailyn, 1993; Burack, 1993). Mechanistic organizations tend to perpetuate the status quo (Pfeffer, 1981), again reducing the likelihood that more senior minority individuals will be available as mentors and potentially limiting minority individuals' access to mentors (cf. Ragins, 1997). Additionally, such organizations often engender a sense of powerlessness among faculty members, threatening the success of faculty at all levels (Lowenstein, Fernandez, & Crane, 2007).

Organizational culture may also have an effect on the mentoring relationship. Monolithic organizations that do not value diversity, but instead emphasize in word and/or deed homogeneity, conformity, assimilation, structural segregation, and the segregation of informal networks are less likely to promote mentoring relationships involving minorities. In contrast, organizations characterized as multicultural value diversity, support mutual accommodation and the preservation of group identities, and use a pluralistic approach (Cox, 1991). It has been suggested that the organizational climate found in multicultural organizations is significantly more conducive to and supportive of mentoring relationships involving minorities, compared to those organizations characterized as monolithic.

Research has also identified a number of obstacles that commonly inhibit institutional efforts to create and sustain a culture of mentoring. These include dissonance between institutional priorities, such as research and clinical productivity; an unwillingness to recognize the amount of time and energy to provide mentoring; and the failure to provide resources adequate to support these demands (Ponce, Williams, & Allen, 2005). There may be additional impediments due to the institution's demands for the creation and maintenance of an institutional culture that supports continuous growth and mastery as reflected, for example, in mentoring and faculty development programs, while simultaneously encouraging competition, independence, and autonomy among faculty and valuing basic science research and clinical research above teaching and faculty development (Ponce et al., 2005; Ramani, 2006).

Several organizational practices have been found to facilitate the success of mentoring programs. The reward of mentors through increased visibility and organizational recognition, such as a banquet, a token gift, or a personal note of appreciation from higher-ranking individuals may encourage mentors to continue their efforts and motivate others to become mentors (Gerstein, 1985). The inclusion of the managers or supervisors of mentors in the process may also increase the likelihood of success.

Programmatic Considerations

Program development requires consideration of the program context, infrastructure, structure, and content. The context refers to the institution, the societal context, and the funding environment in which the program is situated. Program infrastructure encompasses such issues as the screening procedures to be used for mentors and mentees, the selection process to be used following the initial screening for mentors and mentees, the number of mentors potentially available, the extent to which mentors receive support and the nature of that support, and the matching process. Issues of structure include the model(s) of mentoring that is(are) to be employed, the length of time that each mentee cohort will participate in the program, the number of mentees in each cohort, and the expected minimum frequency and intensity of mentor–mentee contact. The content of the program necessarily depends on the specific health-related profession and the extent of the mentees' previous academic, clinical, and research experience. Clearly, several of these issues, such as the number of mentors available, the support provided to mentors, and the structure of the program may depend, at least in part, on the extent and duration of funding available to support the establishment and continuation of a mentoring program. As illustrated below in Table 5.1, the development of a mentoring program can be visualized as a logic model, consisting of inputs, such as staff, mentors, materials, space, mentor and mentee selection and training, and ongoing support; activities, meaning the content of the mentoring program; and outputs, or the achievements of the trainees during and after the conclusion of the mentoring process.

Program Infrastructure

As noted above, program infrastructure refers to issues such as the screening procedures to be used for mentors and mentees, the selection process to be used following the initial screening for mentors and mentees, the number of mentors potentially available, the extent to which mentors receive support and the nature of that support, and the matching process. *The procedures for mentor and mentee screening and selection* may be critical to the success of the mentoring program.

It has been suggested that mentors be required to engage in a self-assessment as part of the screening and selection process. That assessment should allow the prospective mentor to rate himself or herself with respect to his or her comfort level providing mentoring in the domains of self-confidence; educational needs; balancing career and personal life;

TABLE 5.1

Logic Model: Development of a Mentoring Program

Planned Work				Intended Results
Resources/Inputs→	Activities→	Outputs→		Immediate, Intermediate, and Long-Term Outcomes
Resources needed to operate your program and conduct activities	To address problem or asset, activities conducted	As a result of activities conducted, evidence of achievement, examples:		As a result of outputs (service delivery), expected changes in target population in specified period(s) of time
• __(number) of mentors available in __ disciplines • Mentoring program coordinator/director • Advisory board composed of community and institutional stakeholders • Office space for program coordinator/director • Necessary supplies and equipment for program, e.g., computer, etc. • Meeting space for mentor and mentee training sessions and advisory board meetings	• Draft position description for program coordinator/director • Initiate recruitment efforts for program coordinator/director • Hire program coordinator/director • Establish linkages with relevant departments and individuals in institution, e.g., Human Resources, diversity program, department chairs, legal counsel • Establish Advisory Board for mentoring program	• Recruitment efforts will be initiated for program coordinator/director within 1 month of position approval • Program coordinator/director will commence related duties upon hiring • Logs, memos, etc. will document meetings with stakeholders and discussions relating to development of various protocols		**Immediate Outcomes** (e.g., Year 1) • In Year 1, [number] mentors will be recruited and trained. • In Year 1, [number] mentees will be recruited into mentoring program. • In Year 1, there will be [number] mentor–mentee matches. • In Year 1, a total of __ mentor training sessions will be conducted. • In Year 1, a total of __ all-mentor–mentee functions will be conducted, e.g., symposia, workshops, etc. **Intermediate Outcomes** (e.g., Years 2–5) • In Year 2, the number of mentors recruited and trained will be increased by __%. • In Year 2, the number of mentees recruited will be increased by __%. • In Year 2, the number of mentor–mentee matches will be increased by __%. • In Year 2, a total of __ mentor training sessions will be conducted. • In Year 2, a total of __ all-mentor–mentee functions will be conducted, e.g., symposia, workshops, etc. • In Year 2, an evaluation will be conducted of Year 1 mentors, mentees, and the program infrastructure and content to inform future years of the program.

- Private meeting room for individual-level discussion
- Funding
- System of incentives/rewards for mentors

- Establish linkages with relevant national, regional, and local organizations that focus on mentoring health professionals, diversity issues
- Develop and disseminate publicity for mentoring program
- Establish mechanism for recruitment and selection of mentors at multiple levels, e.g., junior, senior
- Develop training program for mentors
- Establish mechanism for screening and selection of mentees to participate in program
- In conjunction with identified stakeholders, develop protocol for evaluation of program, mentors, and mentees

- Advisory Board minutes will document participants and dialogue
- Draft of mentor guidebook will be completed and made available to stakeholders for their review and comment

- In Year 3, the number of mentors recruited and trained will be increased by __%.
- In Year 3, the number of mentees recruited will be increased by __%.
- In Year 3, the number of mentor–mentee matches will be increase by __%.
- In Year 3, a total of __mentor training sessions will be conducted.
- In Year 3, a total of __ all-mentor–mentee functions will be conducted, e.g., symposia, workshops, etc.
- In Year 3, the results of the evaluation conducted in Year 2 will be presented formally to stakeholders for review and discussion regarding integration of findings into program processes and content.
- In Year 4, an evaluation will be conducted of Years 1–3 mentors, mentees, and the program infrastructure and content to inform future years of the program.
- In Year 4, the number of mentors recruited and trained will be increased by __%.
- In Year 4, the number of mentors recruited and trained will be increased by __%.
- In Year 4, the number of mentees recruited will be increased by __%.
- In Year 4, the number of mentor–mentee matches will be increase by __%.
- In Year 4, a total of __mentor training sessions will be conducted.
- In Year 4, a total of __ all-mentor–mentee functions will be conducted, e.g., symposia, workshops, etc.
- In Year 4, the results of the Year 3 evaluation will be presented formally to stakeholders for review and discussion regarding integration of findings into program processes and content.

(Continued)

171

TABLE 5.1 (*Continued*)

Logic Model: Development of a Mentoring Program

Planned Work			Intended Results
Resources/Inputs→	Activities→	Outputs→	Immediate, Intermediate, and Long-Term Outcomes
Resources needed to operate your program and conduct activities	To address problem or asset, activities conducted	As a result of activities conducted, evidence of achievement, examples:	As a result of outputs (service delivery), expected changes in target population in specified period(s) of time
	• Develop joint programs for mentors and mentees • Develop guidebook to assist mentors • Develop and pretest procedures for matching mentors and mentees • Engage consultants as needed to provide technical assistance in development of protocols, evaluation methods and/or analysis		• In Year 4, an evaluation will be conducted of Years 1–3 mentors, mentees, and the program infrastructure and content to inform future years of the program. • In Year 4, an evaluation will be conducted of Years 1–3 mentors, mentees, and the program infrastructure and content to inform future years of the program. • In Year 5, the number of mentors recruited and trained will be increased by __%. • In Year 5, the number of mentees recruited will be increased by __%. • In Year 5, the number of mentor–mentee matches will be increase by __%. • In Year 5, a total of __ all-mentor–mentee functions will be conducted, e.g., symposia, workshops, etc. • In Year 5, the results of the Year 4 evaluation will be presented formally to stakeholders for review and discussion regarding integration of findings into program processes and content. • In Year 5, an evaluation will be conducted of Years 1–4 mentors, mentees, and the program infrastructure and content to inform future years of the program.

Statement of Problem: An effective, high-quality formal mentoring program is needed in order to (1) promote the success; (2) maximize the likelihood of promotion and tenure; (3) maximize the organizational commitment; (4) promote retention; and (5) maximize diversity of junior faculty members at the institution.

networking opportunities; career-related advice, such as the academic preparation needed and the nature of a health-related career; academic issues, such as course selection; the impact of minority status (race/ethnicity/religion/sex/gender/sexual orientation) on one's academic and career development; and the provision of support specific to the particular health profession, such as applications for more advanced training and licensure and certification requirements (Cotter et al., 2004).

A number of existing instruments are available to aid in this self-assessment process. Cotter and colleagues (2004) have recommended the Manifest Needs Questionnaire (Steers & Braunstein, 1976) for use by both the mentor and the prospective mentee at the initiation of the process. Another tool that can be used for this self-assessment is the Measuring Mentoring Potential Scale (MMPS), developed by Darling (1984) on the basis of findings from interviews with 50 nurses, 20 physicians, and 80 health care executives over a 2-year period of time. The tool reflects Darling's conclusion that mentors must meet three specific criteria if the relationship is to be successful: attraction, or liking, which must be mutual between the mentor and the mentee at the initiation of the relationship; action, meaning that the mentor has sufficient time and energy to devote to mentoring; and affect, or mutual respect between the mentor and the mentee. The mentor must minimally be able to fulfill three basic roles, each of which corresponds to one of the absolute requirements: inspirer (attraction), investor (action), and supporter (affect). Finally, the mentor must be able to fulfill at least some of seven additional roles: teacher, feedback-giver, eye-opener, door-opener, idea-bouncer, problem solver, and career counselor.

It is particularly important that the mentor assess accurately the extent to which he or she has time to devote to performing mentoring functions. Researchers have consistently found that mentors with clinical responsibilities often face conflicts in meeting the needs of both their patients and their mentees (Gray & Smith, 2000; Neary, Phillips, & Davies, 1994). Other scholars have noted that there is never sufficient time and that the level of the mentor and mentee commitment to the mentoring process is the key to achieving success within the time that is available for mentoring (Shea, 1999; Zachary, 2000). Although scheduling may present difficulties, regular mentor–mentee meetings are associated with the likelihood that the mentor will be effective in helping the mentee to reduce his or her level of stress (Beecroft, Santner, Lacy, Kunzman, & Dorey, 2006). And, although mentors clearly need sufficient flexibility in order to work with each mentee on an individual basis according to the mentee's needs, the establishment of mentor guidelines is advisable and has been found to be helpful (Gould, Kelly, & Goldstone, 2001).

Mentee screening and selection procedures should assess the mentee's goals, expectations, level of responsibility, strengths, and weaknesses

(Kwasik, Fulda, & John P. Isché Library. 2006), level of motivation as it relates to the mentoring program (Pulsford, Boit, & Owen, 2002), and the likelihood that program participation will enhance his or her career skills (cf. Kwasik et al., 2006). Depending upon the particular discipline, and whether the mentoring program is geared to individuals at the graduate, postdoctoral, or junior faculty/clinician level, it may also be important to consider the extent of the prospective mentee's prior research experience; whether that research was conducted in conjunction with faculty, with students, or alone; whether the mentee has ever submitted a grant proposal, manuscript, or conference abstract; and, if so, whether the grant was funded and/or the manuscript or abstract was accepted.

Three highly divergent strategies have been identified to guide the selection of mentees, each with accompanying benefits and disadvantages. Elite mentoring refers to the selection of an elite cadre of investigators who have already experienced some career successes (Kahn & Greenblatt, 2009). This strategy is likely to be highly successful in terms of mentee success, and is likely to require fewer resources. Because of the "elite" status of the mentee participants, selection to the program may become highly coveted. However, this approach is unlikely to increase the diversity of mentees and may ultimately have less impact because the selected mentees would have been likely to succeed regardless of the mentoring.

In contrast, the selection of struggling investigators who have not had such successes and may not value or even understand the mentoring process would focus resources in individuals who might be considered to be "at risk." However, participation may then be viewed as stigmatizing because selection is limited to those "in trouble." Further, success using this approach is likely to be lower.

Open mentoring offers a third approach to mentee selection. This would ensure that every individual interested in having a mentor would be assigned to one. Because of the wide variability in potential mentees' needs, such a program would require a significant degree of flexibility and the ability to tailor the components to each mentee's needs (Kahn & Greenblatt, 2009).

Mentor–mentee matching in formal mentoring programs is frequently done randomly by third parties, such as a human resources department. Such efforts have been likened to blind dating:

> A current practice of random assignment of protégés to mentors is analogous to blind dates; there would be small probability that the match would be successful, but more attention to the selection phase would raise the probability above chance levels. (Chao, Walz, & Gardner, 1992, p. 634)

Indeed, inappropriate matching has been identified as one of the major reasons for the failure of a mentoring program (Hale, 2000).

Although some writers have advocated as an alternative to random assignment that mentors and mentees participating in a formal mentoring program mutually select each other (Tracy, Jagsi, Starr, & Tarbell, 2004), others have suggested that matching be conducted only after careful consideration of various factors. These include (1) whether to match on the basis of gender, culture, educational level, background, race, ethnicity, age, and/or sexual orientation; (previously addressed in Chapter 4); (2) the extent to which the mentee needs support and/or challenge, recognizing that both are needed to some degree; (3) the extent to which the mentor should also serve as a role model with respect to particular characteristics; (4) the degree of similarity or difference in work styles between the prospective mentor and the prospective mentee; and (5) the degree of congruence in instructional style of the prospective mentor and the learning style of the prospective mentee (Hay, 1995).

Despite its importance, consideration of learning style is frequently neglected in published reports of mentoring programs established for students and faculty in health-related professions. Learning styles are thought of as

> distinctive behaviors which serve as indicators of how a person learns from and adapts to his environment. It also gives clues as to how a person's environment operates. (Gregorc, 1979, p. 234)

> "accessibility characteristics" that provide keys to working more effectively with students . . . interest in learning style focuses on a neglected aspect of individual difference. Knowing about learning-style differences also suggests to the practitioner the most appropriate instructional approach. (Hunt, 1981, p. 647)

> personally preferred way[s] of dealing with information and experience for learning that [cross] content areas. (Della-Dora & Blanchard, 1979, p. 22)

> cognitive, affective, and psychological behaviors that serve as the relatively stable indicators of how learners perceive, interact with, and respond to the learning environment. (Keefe, 1982, p. 44)

Research suggests that culture may have an impact on the general tendencies of individuals' learning style. As an example, Chinese learners have been found to prefer memorization over intuition as a learning strategy, to be more reflective than impulsive, and to have a strong visual orientation (Kennedy, 2002).

The term "learning style" is frequently used interchangeably with the term "cognitive style." Cassidy (2004, pp. 420–421) distinguished between the two, explaining that the term cognitive style refers to

> an individual's typical or habitual mode of problem solving, thinking, perceiving and remembering, while the term learning style is adopted to reflect a concern with the application of cognitive style in a learning situation.

Cognitive style has also been conceived of as an individual's consistent approach to the processing and organization of information (Messick, 1984; Tennant, 1988). As such, cognitive style represents a significant component of learning style.

Similarities in cognitive style between members of a dyad are believed to lead to smoother interactions, mutuality of positive feelings (Triandis, 1960; Witkin, Moore, Goodenough, & Cox, 1977), more effective communication (Frank & Davis, 1982), greater satisfaction with the relationship (Cooper & Miller, 1991), and similar perceptions of the relationship (Handley, 1982). A study involving 53 mentor–protégé dyads, including physicians, found that similarities in cognitive style were also associated with more career and psychosocial functions reported within the mentoring relationship (Armstrong, Allinson, & Hayes, 2002). Dissimilar cognitive styles within the dyad may be associated with increased levels of frustration and conflict (Mumford, 1995; Witkin & Goodenough, 1981).

Prospective mentors and mentees may actually be unaware of how they teach and learn, respectively. A self-assessment on the basis of one of the numerous models that have been developed to understand and to portray the various strategies used in the process of learning may be critical to the selection of trainees for a specific program or the design of a program to meet the needs of various trainees (Honey & Mumford, 1983). A study involving 200 health professionals, including nurses, pharmacists, dietitians, and physiotherapists, found that learning was most likely to occur when the clinicians participated in activities that were congruent with their learning style (Currie, 1995). Another study concluded that medical students' learning and attitudes are likely to improve if the learning tasks and teaching methods are adapted to their learning styles and preferences (Chapman & Calhoun, 2006).

Three models of learning that are frequently used as the basis for the development of teaching approaches include Curry's Onion Model (Curry, 1983, 1987), Kolb's Experiential Model of Information Processing (Kolb, 1976, 1984; Kolb, Rubin, & McIntyre, 1974), and Honey and Mumford's Model of Experiential Learning (Honey & Mumford, 1992; Mumford, 1995). Table 5.2 provides an outline of the key features of each of these models.

Program Structure

The structure of the mentoring program necessarily depends on the available infrastructure to support it. As an example, a multiple mentoring model may be preferred but this option is foreclosed if there is an inadequate number of faculty available to serve as mentors and e-mentoring is unavailable to extend the mentoring network. A program of shorter length, such as a summer institute, is less costly, but is likely of too short a duration to transform mentees into independent researchers; at most, it may serve as a vehicle to stimulate interest in health research as a career.

TABLE 5.2

Structure and Features of Three Models of Learning

Model	Structure	Key Features
Curry's Onion Model (Curry, 1983, 1987)	Four-layer model: *Instructional process*: outermost layer representing preferred mode of learning in specific situations *Social interaction*: refers to individual's preference relating to social interaction during learning process *Information process style*: how individuals assimilate information through orienting, sensory loading, short-term memory, enhanced association, coding, and long-term storage *Cognitive personality style*: innermost layer referring to how individuals adapt information as it has been assimilated through information processing style	Level of stability increases and susceptibility to external events decreases from the outermost layer or process to the innermost layer
Kolb's Experiential Model of Information Processing (Kolb, 1976, 1984; Kolb, Rubin, & McIntyre, 1974)	Individuals process information through four modes that exist along two orthogonal dimensions: Abstract Conceptualization–Concrete Experience and Active Experimentation–Reflective Observation These yield four learning styles: *Converger*: relies on abstract conceptualization and active experimentation *Diverger*: uses concrete experience and reflective observation *Assimilator*: relies upon abstract conceptualization and reflective observation *Accommodator*: uses concrete experience and active experimentation	Conceives of learning as a cyclical process consisting of concrete experience, observations and reflection, the formation of abstract concepts and generalizations, and the testing of resulting implications in new situations

(Continued)

TABLE 5.2 (Continued)

Structure and Features of Three Models of Learning

Model	Structure	Key Features
Honey and Mumford's Model of Experiential Learning (Honey & Mumford, 1992; Mumford, 1995)	Four types of learners: *Activists:* willing to try anything once, appreciate the challenge presented by new experiences; frequently engage with other people; bored with long-term consolidation *Reflectors:* collect and analyze data before drawing conclusions; consider all perspectives before making a decision or pursuing a course of action; more likely to observe others in action than to take an active role in meetings *Theorists:* focus on theories, models, and systems; value rationality and logic; dislike ambiguity; tend to be analytical and detached *Pragmatists:* view problems as challenges; actively pursue new solutions or techniques that may be useful in a specific situation; eager to experiment	Each experiential learning style reflects a particular stage in the learning cycle. The activist corresponds to having an experience, the reflector to reviewing the experience, the theorist concludes from the experience, and the pragmatist focuses on the planning of the next steps to be taken.

Nevertheless, successful mentoring programs for health professionals have relied on a variety of different structures. As an example, the University of California, San Diego has developed a short term, intensive mentoring program to train students at varying levels of education and experience in research in geriatric psychiatry (Halpain, Jeste, Katz, & Lebowitz, 1997; Halpain et al., 2001; Halpain, Trinidad, Wetherell, Lebowitz, & Jeste, 2005). In contrast, Case Western Reserve University has developed a year-long training program for international mentees in international research ethics that encompasses substantive training in the field of research ethics, career mentoring, and psychosocial mentoring. Although the substantive portion of the training program is approximately 1-year in length, the mentoring functions are available to mentees for several years, while they are in the United States and following their return to their home countries.

Program structure must also consider the mentoring and teaching approaches to be used in the program. These may include one or more of the following: small group teaching, real or simulated case studies, experiential learning, didactic teaching, problem-based learning, self-directed work, role playing, mentee teaching opportunities, self-directed research, and/or videos (Cooper, Carlisle, Gibbs, & Watkins, 2001; cf. Sadler-Smith & Riding, 1999). The specific approaches to be used may be dependent upon the mentee's then-current stage of learning and the specific focus of the interaction. As an example, small group teaching may be an effective approach to working with mentees to develop skills in manuscript preparation, but role playing may be more appropriate to enhance mentee efforts in securing an academic appointment following completion of a PhD degree. Ideally, the teaching approaches used should be selected for their congruence with the mentees' learning styles in order to maximize the benefit to the mentees.

Program Content

As indicated, the specific program content may depend to some degree on the specific health-related career for which the mentee is being trained and his or her level of education and experience prior to initiation of the mentoring relationship. However, regardless of the specific career, the mentoring program should address both career and psychosocial functions. Suggested components of each of these functions are noted in Table 5.3.

As indicated in Chapter 1, focusing on the process and models of mentoring, the duration of a mentoring relationship may vary across mentees due to differences in their level of experience at the commencement of the mentoring relationship. Program content should be organized in such a way that it considers the differing levels of mentees' need and the varying lengths of the mentoring relationships.

TABLE 5.3

Content of Career and Psychosocial Mentoring

Career Functions	Psychosocial Functions
Teaching approaches	Balancing career and family
Grant writing	Stress management
Grant management	
Manuscript preparation	
Budgeting	
Teamwork	
Conflict management	
Communication	
Negotiation skills	
Time management	
Development of networks	
Research and/or clinical ethics	
Guidance in acquiring necessary professional licensure or certification	
Self-promotion	

Compiled from Bickel, 1995; Wright-Harp & Cole, 2008.

Academic institutions and other entities may wish to consider providing prospective employees or students with career and/or psychosocial mentoring even prior to the individual's formal application for employment or admission. A study of the relationship between psychosocial and career mentoring and organizational attractiveness conducted with European graduate students found that prehire psychosocial mentoring provided by a company was associated with an increase in the students' interest in prospective employment with the company (Spitzmüller, et al., 2008). The provision of accurate information about the organization and what would be required to succeed appeared to discourage some applicants, but may have resulted in a better alignment, or fit, between those who did apply and the organizational environment. This may be particularly critical in an institution's efforts to attract specific students or faculty members to the institution.

Mentor Training

The foundation of mentor training is to define the role of the mentor and its associated expectations. A written job description provided to be the mentor and mentee can be used to apprise both of the parameters of the relationship. However, sufficient flexibility must also be maintained to permit creativity (Gerstein, 1985).

Although lectures and seminars are frequently used to train mentors, research indicates that this may not be effective in comparison with other approaches, such as critical reflection and experiential learning (Garvey & Alred, 2000). It has been suggested that, above all else, mentor training must focus on strategies to promote the development of the mentees (Ramanan, Phillips, Davis, Silen, & Reede, 2002). The content of the mentor training should address communication, coaching, socialization of newcomers, and issues related to career progression. All mentors should receive training and support in how to address issues of diversity and discrimination. Training in additional areas may be necessary depending upon the mentoring model that is to be used. For example, if mentor–mentee communication will include e-mentoring, it will be important to verify that the prospective mentor has adequate computer skills and to provide training to those prospective mentors who do not.

Research findings raise the possibility that mentors may be unable to adequately counsel their mentees with respect to clinical and research ethics because of their own inadequate knowledge and understanding. Researchers conducting a survey of a national random sample of 195 university health education faculty in graduate level programs, almost all of whom had presented their research at professional conferences or published their research in professional journals, found that the majority of respondents characterized three scenarios as ethical that involved ethically questionable conduct (Price, Dake, & Islam, 2001). Scholars in several disciplines have noted this deficiency among mentors and have urged the adoption of mentor-centered ethics training to enable mentors to more fully develop their ethical reasoning capabilities and as a prelude working with mentees (Brown, Daly, & Leong, 2009; Motta, 2002).

Various health science institutions have developed mentoring programs that offer excellent resources. The University of California San Francisco's *Mentoring Toolkit* (2007) delineates the roles and expectations of the mentor and the mentee; provides a Mentoring Partnership Agreement that commits the mentor and mentee to abide by specified guidelines; and furnishes checklists that may be helpful in establishing the parameters of the mentoring relationship, such as the frequency of meetings and mechanism for exchange of feedback.

A tiered approach to mentoring may be helpful to newly recruited, inexperienced mentors. This approach would recruit more senior individuals who have track records of successfully mentoring more junior faculty and clinical professionals to mentor more junior faculty or professionals in their efforts to mentor individuals who are even more junior. For example, a junior faculty member who has no previous experience in mentoring but has published extensively and who has a record of successfully competing for research grants may wish to mentor a PhD student. A more senior faculty member who has successfully mentored other junior faculty in their career development may mentor the junior faculty member in his or her efforts to mentor the graduate student.

Mentee Training

Relatively little literature has focused on training or preparation for the mentee role. As noted in Chapter 1, a variety of instruments are available to assist mentees in the identification of their strengths and weakness. (See Chapter 1 for a brief listing.)

Although an assessment of strengths and weakness will help to lay the groundwork, it is not by itself adequate preparation for a mentoring relationship. Mentee training should ideally address the nature of a mentoring relationship; expectations of mentors and mentees in terms of meetings, time commitment, functions, and so on; approaches to conflict resolution and potential difficulties and strategies to overcome them; and available resources in the event that difficulties in the mentoring relationship do arise. Depending upon the program structure, mentee training may also encompass factors to consider in selecting a mentor; and benefits and drawbacks to various models of mentoring that may be relevant, for example, whether to have one or several mentors.

EVALUATION

The Institutional Environment

Relatively little has been published regarding evaluations of the institutional environment vis-à-vis the effectiveness or efficiency of mentoring programs. Factors to be considered include the extent of structural segregation, the existence and nature of rewards to faculty for providing mentoring; the ability to recruit mentors within the institution, and institutional success in establishing and sustaining formal mentoring programs through the receipt of government or foundation training grants.

Program Success

Scholars have delineated five elements that comprise the quality of a program in higher education: (1) excellence, meaning that something is exceptional; (2) perfection, referring to the consistency of quality; (3) fit for purpose, that is, the quality fulfills a specific purpose as perceived by stakeholders; (4) value for money, so that the benefit is optimal relative to the cost; and (5) transformation, whereby the quality both empowers and enhances the learner (Harvey & Green, 1993; Lomas, 2002). Others have advocated the elimination of the quality of perfection from this matrix, noting that higher education does not aim to produce cloned graduates (Watty, 2003). Because mentoring programs focus on the personal and professional transformation of the mentee (Miller, 2002), it has been suggested that program evaluation should assess, in particular, the extent to which mentees have been transformed, enhanced, and empowered (McMillan & Parker, 2005). This presents significant challenges because such constructs are not easily measured.

Accordingly, evaluation of a mentoring program requires that the inquiry examine program structures, mechanisms, and procedures (Harvey & Newton, 2004) and follow a cyclical pattern of action and reflection, so that the results of the evaluative process are then used to effectuate improvements; evaluation, then, is a continuous, iterative process. Although speaking of teaching, the conceptualization of this cycle by Ashcroft and Palacio (1996) is relevant to the evaluation of a mentoring program:

> We have conceptualized reflective action in teaching as an evaluation-led activity in which evaluation and the collection of data about the context for action leads to reflection on the significance of that data, and that in turn informs planning, provision and action. On the completion of this cycle, evaluation again takes place, this time into effectiveness of action, leading to another cycle of reflection, planning and action. (Ashcroft & Palacio, 1996, p. 94)

This comprehensive evaluation of the mentoring program requires an assessment of both what is happening in the program and why it is happening, suggesting that both quantitative and qualitative approaches are needed for a comprehensive evaluation (Biggs, 2000; McMillan & Parker, 2005). Table 5.4 provides an outline of the constructs to be assessed, potential measures of these constructs, and sources of the data for that portion of the evaluation.

It is worth noting that few of the published reports of mentoring programs' effectiveness include an examination of the financial costs associated with the program or the efficiency of the program, that is, the cost effectiveness or the ratio between the dollars expended and the program's success (Buddeberg-Fischer & Herta, 2006). One exception is the report of the National Center of Leadership in Academic Medicine of the University of California, San Diego, which presented data on the cost benefit of their mentoring program (Wingard, Garman, & Reznik, 2004). Researchers calculated the return-on-investment using the following formula:

$$\frac{(\text{Total benefits} - \text{Total costs})}{\text{Total costs}} \times 100$$

TABLE 5.4
Constructs, Measures, and Sources of Data for Mentoring Program Evaluation

Construct	Measure	Sources of Data
Excellence	Quality of mentors	Mentee survey/questionnaire Mentee interview
Fit for purpose	Length of program Minimum acceptable frequency of mentor–mentee interaction Minimum acceptable intensity of mentor–mentee interaction Technology used	Mentor/mentee survey/questionnaires Mentor/mentee interviews/focus groups Non-mentor faculty input
Value for money	Quality of mentees applying Mentee completion rate Financial cost of program Financial return to program Nonfinancial costs of program Nonfinancial return to program, e.g., status	Applicant portfolios Graduation rate of student mentees Mentee financial contributions to institution and/or program Mentee loyalty to institution or program, e.g., attendance at events, public relations efforts Attainment of promotion and tenure for faculty mentees
Transformation	Improvement in mentee self-efficacy Increase in mentee skills	Mentee questionnaires/interviews Mentee productivity, e.g., grants, publications

Derived in part from: Buddeberg-Fischer & Herta, 2006; Harvey & Green, 1993; Lomas, 2002; Stewart, 2009; Watty, 2003.

Program cost was calculated based on these expenses: for each participating junior faculty member, salary reimbursement to departments, operational program costs, and a stipend provided to each mentor. These costs were compared to the estimated savings that accrued through improved retention rates of the mentored faculty that resulted in decreased costs of recruitment.

Mentor Functions

Scholars have noted the absence of specific benchmarks for the evaluation of mentors and have advocated their delineation (Opipari-Arrigan, Stark, & Drotar, 2005; Rosenthal & Black, 2006). Noe (1988) suggested that an evaluation of the mentor encompass an assessment of his or her performance in eight mentor domains: acceptance and confirmation, challenging assignments, coaching, counseling, exposure and visibility, friendship, role model, and sponsorship. Accordingly, Noe developed a 29-item scale to be completed by the mentee that assesses the extent to which the mentor fulfilled these functions. However, the extent to which these domains have been addressed can also be evaluated through reliance on instruments in addition to a questionnaire or survey of the mentee. Noe's eight domains are used in Table 5.5 in order to illustrate the various aspects of the mentoring function that fall within each such domain and the tools that can be potentially used for their evaluation.

As the table indicates, reliance on both quantitative and qualitative assessment tools is recommended. Surveys and questionnaires used for evaluations of mentors, mentees, and mentoring programs often use Likert scales as a means of collecting quantitative data. Additional quantitative data can be obtained through the use of mentee diaries, field notes, and CVs, in which he or she has recorded meetings, presentations, conferences, and so forth. Mentee field notes and diaries can also provide qualitative data. One technique that appears to be less used but that may be valuable in the context of evaluation is the critical incident technique (Flanagan, 1954). This strategy consists of paired questions that are used to probe for positive and negative experiences. This technique is more likely than open-ended questioning to elicit specific comments from the respondents, which can then be analyzed qualitatively for themes.

Mentee Success

Mentee success has traditionally been assessed based on whether specified "benchmarks" have been attained. These are achievements that can be quantified, such as the number of publications and the number of presentations at professional conferences. Mentees' career trajectory, assessed on position title, salary, rank, and level of responsibility, has also been used as a measure of success. Table 5.5 lists many of these benchmarks and potential sources from which these data can be derived.

Mentee self-reports are often used to assess mentees' level of career satisfaction and self-efficacy. These assessments commonly rely on a Likert scale. As seen in Table 5.6, mentee narratives can also be used; these are likely to yield more detailed information than a Likert scale would, but the data entry and analysis associated with narratives are significantly more time- and labor-intensive.

Relatively few published reports reflect long-term follow-up of mentees. Indeed, apart from funded training programs that require long-term follow-up of trainees in order to establish effectiveness and sustainability of efforts, many programs may be tempted to forego this task because of

TABLE 5.5

Criteria and Measures of Mentor Excellence

Function	Domain	Measure	Source of Data
Career mentoring	Challenging assignments	Introduces mentee to new ideas Shares relevant information with mentee Engages in discussion Sets high standards Presents opportunities to learn new skills	Mentee questionnaire/ survey Mentee interview Presentations at/ submission to professional meetings Mentee field notes or diary Critical incident account
	Coaching	Discusses career plans Acts as sounding board for ideas Suggests alternative means of performing a task or accomplishing a goal Stimulates critical thinking Gives positive feedback Enhances mentee confidence Encourages mentee independence	Mentee questionnaire/ survey Mentee interview Mentee field notes or diary Critical incident account
	Exposure and visibility	Facilitates communication between mentee and clients/patients/ colleagues Introduces mentee to colleagues Promotes mentee's visibility	Mentee questionnaire/ survey Mentee interview Mentee field notes or diary Critical incident account
	Protection	Advocates on behalf of mentee Provides structure	Mentee questionnaire/ survey Mentee interview Mentee field notes or diary Critical incident account

Function	Domain	Measure	Source of Data
	Role model	Acts as a role model	Mentee questionnaire/ survey Mentee interview Mentee field notes or diary Critical incident account
	Sponsorship	Provides opportunities for collaboration	Mentee questionnaire/ survey Mentee interview Mentee field notes or diary Critical incident account Published manuscripts with mentee as author
Psychosocial mentoring	Counseling	Sensitive to mentee's personal needs Assists mentee with family-work balance Provides mentee with emotional support Helps reduce stress Actively listens Maintains confidentiality Motivates mentee to accept challenges	Mentee questionnaire/ survey Mentee interview Mentee field notes or diary Critical incident account
	Acceptance and confirmation	Treats mentee with respect	Mentee questionnaire/ survey Mentee interview Mentee field notes or diary Critical incident account
	Friendship	Invites mentee to participate in social activities	Mentee questionnaire/ survey Mentee interview Mentee field notes or diary Critical incident account

Derived from: Beecroft, Santner, Lacy, Kunzman, & Dorey, 2006; Burke, McKeen, & McKenna, 1994; Daloz, 1986; Erdem & Aytemur, 2008; Noe, 1988; Ragins & McFarkin, 1990; Suen & Chow, 2001.

TABLE 5.6
Criteria and Measures of Mentee Success

Criterion	Measure	Source of Data	Approach
Academic achievement	Completion of program Grade point average	Academic record	Academic record at institution Long-term follow-up of mentee's academic career
External recognition	Professional award	Mentee self-report Professional publications	Mentee questionnaire/ survey
Career trajectory	Position and rank Salary Level of professional responsibility Grant funding Publication/ presentation record	Mentee self-report Funding agency databases Research databases	Mentee questionnaire/ survey Web search
Self-efficacy	Self-assessment	Mentee self-report	Mentee questionnaire/ survey Mentee self-assessment Mentee diary/field notes
Career commitment	Mentee career trajectory	Mentee self-report Longitudinal follow-up of mentee	Mentee questionnaire/ survey Mentee interview at program completion Periodic questionnaire of mentee over time

Compiled from Cooper, Carlisle, Gibbs, & Watkins, 2001; Girves, Zepeda, & Gwathmey, 2005; Gray & Smith, 1999; Hurst & Koplin-Baucum, 2005.

the time and labor required for follow-up. Mentees often move following completion of their training and they may move several times. Although they may have an interest in remaining in touch with their mentor, they may have little incentive to maintain communication with an institution in which a formal mentoring program is housed if their mentor should leave. This underscores the need to develop a triadic mentoring relationship comprised of the sponsoring institution, the mentor, and the mentee. The development of mentee programmatic and institutional bonds may be critical to both the ability to evaluate mentee long-term success and the effectiveness of the program and institution over time.

The Mentor–Mentee Relationships

Evaluation of the mentor–mentee relationship should not be confused with an evaluation of the extent to which either the mentor or the mentee fulfilled their responsibilities, such as having meetings or engaging in dialogue. Rather, it is an evaluation of the interaction and the dynamic between them: the purposefulness of the meetings, the quality of the dialogue, and the quality of their engagement in the mentoring process (Detsky & Baerlocher, 2007). Ideally, this assessment should be conducted longitudinally during the course of the relationship, rather than at a single point in time during the relationship, or following the termination of the mentoring relationship (Walker et al., 2002). An evaluation while the relationship is ongoing provides the mentee and mentor with an opportunity for course correction and, if the situation so warrants, early termination of the relationship (Detsky & Baerlocher, 2007). Table 5.7 provides criteria and measures that can be used for this evaluation, as well as potential sources for these data.

Berk and colleagues (2005) developed the Mentorship Effectiveness Scale to assess from the mentee's perspective the extent to which the mentor fulfilled his or her responsibilities (e.g., "My mentor suggested appropriate resources") as well as various aspects of the mentor–mentee

TABLE 5.7
Criteria and Measures of Mentoring Relationship

Criterion	Measure	Source of Data
Consistency	Mutuality of respect	Mentee questionnaire/survey Mentor questionnaire/survey
Availability	Mutuality of effort to be available for mentoring	Mentee questionnaire/survey Mentor questionnaire/survey Mentor field notes Mentee field notes
Communication	Mutuality of communication efforts Mutual sharing of experiences and opportunities	Mentee questionnaire/survey Mentor questionnaire/survey
Fairness/justice	Mutual contribution to mentoring relationship Acknowledgment of contributions by each Shared control Mutuality of trust	Mentee questionnaire/survey Mentor questionnaire/survey

Sources: Erdem & Aytemur, 2008; McAllister, Ahmedani, Harold, & Cramer, 2009; Stewart, 2009.

relationship (e.g., "My mentor was approachable"). However, the absence of a mentor's evaluation of the relationship ultimately limits the usefulness of the instrument as a starting point for the improvement of the mentoring relationship and places all of the responsibility for the effectiveness of the relationship on the mentor.

Cotter and colleagues (2004) have suggested the use of specific instruments for the evaluation of a mentoring relationship, to be completed by both the mentor and the mentee at the conclusion of the mentoring program. These include: Orientation to Relationships (Lahiri, 2000), Professional Commitment (Mowday, Steers, & Porter, 1979), Career Expectations (Scandura & Schriesheim, 1991), and Expected Costs and Benefits to Being a Mentor (Ragins & Scandura, 1999). Allinson and colleagues (2001) proposed that the degree to which mentor–mentee contact results in idea generation also be used as a tool in assessing the relationship, noting that ultimately the extent of idea generation serves as a measure of productivity within the relationship. Other scholars have also suggested that the relationship be evaluated for the degree of similarity between the mentee and the mentor participating in a formal mentoring program (Armstrong et al., 2002). However, this suggests that a goal of the mentoring program should be the development of mentees who are similar to their mentors. This may implicitly discourage the selection of mentees from sexual, racial, or ethnic minority groups.

The success of the mentoring relationship with respect to junior faculty members and beginning clinicians can also be evaluated through an assessment of the mentee's organization commitment and citizenship behavior. Research outside of the context of the health professions suggests that informal mentoring relationships perceived by mentees as high in quality are associated with increased levels of organizational commitment and organizational citizenship behavior (Donaldson, Ensher, & Grant-Vallone, 2000). Organizational commitment is defined as the strength of an individual's identification and involvement in his or her organization (Mowday, Porter, & Steers, 1982; Mowday et al., 1979). Organizational citizenship behavior refers to behavior that is discretionary and that represents what would normally be expected in the context of satisfactory job performance, such as assisting coworkers to resolve a problem (Mackenzie, Podsakoff, & Fetter, 1993; Organ & Konovsky, 1989; Organ & Ryan, 1995; Podsakoff, MacKenzie, & Hui, 1993).

SUMMARY

Mentoring, regardless of the model used, is enormously complex; numerous factors must be considered in the development of formal mentoring programs and the evaluation of both formal and informal mentoring.

Consideration must be given to the context (e.g., organizational setting and available funding), infrastructure (screening procedures for mentors and mentees, the matching process, etc.), structure (model, duration, intensity, teaching approaches), and content of the program (mentor and mentee training).

The evaluation process must consider each level of the mentoring process: the institutional, programmatic, mentor, mentee, and mentor–mentee relationship. Both quantitative and qualitative tools are available to aid in this assessment. Few reports have provided details on the institutional context in which programs are situated and the relationship between that context and program success. Although published reports often highlight the program successes, the majority of these reports focus on short-term findings and fail to follow programs, mentors or mentees longitudinally. Evaluations focusing on the financial costs and benefits of formal mentoring programs in the health professions are similarly few. These gaps in the literature underscore the need for additional research into factors associated with successful mentoring and the extent to which the benefits of mentoring gained by institutions, programs, mentors, and mentees are sustained over time.

REFERENCES

Allinson, C. W., Armstrong, S. J., & Hayes, J. (2001). The effect of cognitive style on leader-member exchange: A study of manager-subordinate dyads. *Journal of Occupational and Organizational Psychology, 74,* 201–220.

Armstrong, S. J., Allinson, C. W., & Hayes, J. (2002). Formal mentoring systems: An examination of the effects of mentor/protégé cognitive styles of the mentoring process. *Journal of Management Studies, 39*(8), 1111–1137.

Ashcroft, K., & Palacio, D. (1996). *Researching into assessment and evaluation in colleges and universities.* London: Tavistock.

Bailyn, L. (1993). *Breaking the mold: Women, men, and time in the new corporate world.* New York: The Free Press.

Beecroft, P. C., Santner, S., Lacy, M. L., Kunzman, L., & Dorey, F. (2006). New graduate nurses' perceptions of mentoring: Six-year programme evaluation. *Journal of Advanced Nursing, 55*(6), 736–747.

Berk, R. A., Berg, J., Mortimer, R., Walton-Moss, B., & Yeo, T. P. (2005). Measuring the effectiveness of faculty mentoring relationships. *Academic Medicine, 80*(1), 66–71.

Bickel, J. (1995). Scenarios for success—Enhancing women physicians' professional advancement. *Western Journal of Medicine, 162,* 165–169.

Brown, R. T., Daley, B. P., & Leong, F. T. L. (2009). Mentoring in research: A developmental approach. *Professional Psychology, Research, and Practice, 40*(3), 306–313.

Buddeberg-Fischer, B., & Herta, K-D. (2006). Formal mentoring programmes for medical students and doctors—A review of the Medline literature. *Medical Teacher, 28*(3), 248–257.

Burack, E. H. (1993). *Corporate resurgence and the new employment relationships: After the reckoning.* Westport, CT: Quorum.

Burke, R. J., McKeen, C. A., & McKenna, C. (1994). Benefits of mentoring in organizations: The mentors perspective. *Journal of Managerial Psychology, 19*(3), 23–32.

Burns, T., & Stalker, G. M. (1961). *The management of innovation.* London: Tavistock.

Cassidy, S. (2004). Learning styles: An overview of theories, models, and measures. *Educational Psychology, 24*(4), 419–444.

Chao, G. T., Walz, P. M., & Gardner, P. D. (1992). Formal and informal mentorships: A comparison on mentoring functions and contrast with non-mentored counterparts. *Personnel Psychology, 45,* 619–636.

Chapman, D. M., & Calhoun, J. G. (2006). Validation of learning style measures: Implications for medical education practice. *Medical Education, 40,* 576–583.

Cooper, H., Carlisle, C., Gibbs, T., & Watkins, C. (2001). Developing an evidence base for interdisciplinary learning: A systematic review. *Journal of Advanced Nursing, 35*(2), 228–237.

Cooper, S. E., & Miller, J. A. (1991). MBTI learning style-teaching style discongruences. *Educational and Psychological Measurement, 51,* 699–706.

Cotter, J. J., Coogle, C. L., Parham, I. A., Head, C., Fulton, L., Watson, K., et al. (2004). Designing a multi-disciplinary geriatrics health professional mentoring program. *Educational Gerontology, 30,* 107–117.

Cox, T. (1991). The multicultural organization. *Academy of Management Executive, 5*(2), 34–47.

Cox, T. (1993). *Cultural diversity in organizations: Theory, research, and practice.* San Francisco: Berret-Koehler.

Currie, G. (1995). Learning theory and the design of training in a health authority. *Health Manpower Management, 21*(2), 13–19.

Curry, L. (1983). *An organisation of learning styles theory and construct.* ERIC document no. ED 235 185.

Curry, L. (1987). *Integrating concepts of cognitive or learning style: A review with attention to psychometric standards.* Ottawa, ON Canada: Canadian College of Health Service Executives.

Daloz, L. A. (1986). *Effective teaching and mentoring: Realizing the transformational power of adult learning experiences.* San Francisco: Jossey-Bass.

Darling, L. A. (1984). What do nurses want in a mentor? *Journal of Nursing Administration, 14,* 42–44.

Della-Dora, D., & Blanchard, L. J. (1979). *Moving toward self-directed learning: Highlights of relevant research and promising practice.* Alexandria, VA: Association for Supervision and Curriculum Development.

Detsky, A. S., & Baerlocher, M. O. (2007). Academic mentoring—How to give it and how to get it. *Journal of the American Medical Association, 297*(19), 2134–2136.

Donaldson, S. I., Ensher, E. A., & Grant-Vallone, E. J. (2000). Longitudinal examination of mentoring relationships on organizational commitment and citizenship behavior. *Journal of Career Development, 26*(4), 233–249.

Erdem, F., & Aytemur, J. O. (2008). Mentoring—A relationship based on trust: Qualitative research. *Public Personnel Management, 37*(1), 55–65.

Flanagan, J. C. (1954). The critical incident technique. *Psychological Bulletin, 51,* 327–358.

Frank, B. M., & Davis, J. K. (1982). Effect of field-independence match or mismatch on a communication task. *Journal of Educational Psychology, 74,* 23–31.

Garvey, B., & Alred, G. (2000). Developing mentors. *Career Development International, 5,* 216–222.

Gerstein, M. (1985). Mentoring: An age old practice in a knowledge-based society. *Journal of Counseling and Development, 64,* 156–157.

Girves, J. E., Zepeda, Y., & Gwathmey, J. K. (2005). Mentoring in a post-affirmative action world. *Journal of Social Issues, 61*(3), 449–479.

Gould, D., Kelly, D., & Goldstone, L. (2001). Preparing nurse managers to mentor students. *Nursing Standard, 16*(11), 39–42.

Gray, M., & Smith, L. N. (1999). The professional socialization of diploma of higher education in nursing students (Project 2000): A longitudinal qualitative study. *Journal of Advanced Nursing, 29*(3), 639–647.

Gray, M. A., & Smith, L. N. (2000). The qualities of an effective mentor from the student nurse's perspective: Findings from a longitudinal qualitative study. *Journal of Advanced Nursing, 32*(6), 1542–1549.

Gregorc, A. F. (1979). Learning styles: Potent forces behind them. *Educational Leadership, 36*(2), 234–237.

Hale, R. (2000). To match or mis-match? The dynamics of mentoring as a route to personal and organizational learning. *Career Development International, 5,* 223–234.

Halpain, M. C., Jeste, D. V., Katz, I. R., & Lebowitz, B. D. (1997). The first Summer Research Institute in geriatric psychiatry. *American Journal of Geriatric Psychiatry, 5,* 238–246.

Halpain, M. C., Jeste, D. V., Katz, I. R., Reynold, C. F., III., Small, G. W., Borson, S., et al. (2001). Summer Research Institute: Enhancing research career development in geriatric psychiatry. *Academic Psychiatry, 25,* 48–56.

Halpain, M. C., Trinidad, G. I., Wetherell, J. L., Lebowitz, B. D., & Jeste, D. V. (2005). Intensive short-term research training for undergraduate, graduate, and medical students: Early experience with a new national-level approach in geriatric mental health. *Academic Psychiatry, 29,* 58–65.

Handley, P. (1982). Relationship between supervisors' and trainees' cognitive styles and the supervision process. *Journal of Counseling Psychology, 29,* 508–515.

Harvey, L., & Green, D. (1993). Defining quality. *Assessment and Evaluation in Higher Education, 18*(1), 9–34.

Harvey, L., & Newton, J. (2004). Transforming quality evaluation. *Quality in Higher Education, 10*(2), 149–165.

Hay, J. (1995). *Transformational mentoring.* London: McGraw-Hill.

Honey, P., & Mumford, A. (1992). *Manual of learning styles* (3rd ed.). Maidenhead, UK: Honey.

Honey, P., & Mumford, A. (1983). *Using your learning styles.* Maidenhead, UK: Peter Honey Publications.

Hunt, D. E. (1981). Learning style and the interdependence of practice and theory. *Phi Delta Kappan, 62*(9), 647.

Hurst, S. M., & Koplin-Baucum, S. (2005). Mentor program: Evaluation, change, and challenges. *Dimensions of Critical Care Nursing, 24*(6), 273–274.

Kahn, J. S., & Greenblatt, R. M. (2009). Mentoring career scientists for HIV research careers. *American Journal of Public Health, 99*, S37–S42.

Keefe, J. W. (1982). Assessing student learning styles: An overview. In J. W. Keefe (Ed.), *Student learning styles and brain behavior* (pp. 43–53). Reston, VA: National Association of Secondary School Principals.

Kennedy, P. (2002). Learning cultures and learning styles: Myth-understandings about adult (Hong Kong) Chinese learners. *International Journal of Lifelong Education, 21*(3), 430–445.

Kolb, D. A. (1976). Management and learning processes. *California Management Review, 18*(3), 21–31.

Kolb, D. A. (1984). *Experiential learning experience as the source of learning and development.* Englewood Cliffs, NJ: Prentice-Hall.

Kolb, D. A., Rubin, I. M., & McIntyre, J. M. (1974). *Organisational psychology—An experiential approach.* Englewood Cliffs, NJ: Prentice-Hall.

Kwasik, H., Fulda, P. O., & John P. Isché Library. (2006). Strengthening professionals: A chapter-level formative evaluation of the Medical Library Association mentoring initiative. *Journal of the Medical Library Association, 94*(1), 19–29.

Lahiri, I. (2000). *Diversity leader self-assessment.* Workforce Development Group. Retrieved June 2009 from http://www.workforcedevelopmentgroup.com/individual_assess.htm

Lowenstein, S. R., Fernandez, G., & Crane, L. A. (2007). Medical school faculty discontent: Prevalence and predictors of intent to leave academic careers *BMC Medical Education, 7*, 37.

MacKenzie, S. B., Podsakoff, P. M., & Fetter, R. (1993). The impact of organizational citizenship behavior on evaluations of salespersons performance. *Journal of Marketing, 57*, 70–80.

McMillan, W., & Parker, M. E. (2005). 'Quality is bound up with our values': Evaluating the quality of mentoring programmes. *Quality in Higher Education, 11*(2), 151–160.

Messick, S. (1984). The nature of cognitive styles: Problems and promise in educational practice. *Educational Psychologist, 19*(2), 59–74.

Miller, A. (2002). *Mentoring students and young people: A handbook for effective practice.* London: Kogan Page.

Motta, M. M. (2002). Mentoring the mentors: The Yoda factor in promoting scientific integrity. *American Journal of Bioethics, 2*(4), 1–2.

Mowday, R. T., Porter, L. W., & Steers, R. M. (1982). *Employee-organizational linkages: The psychology of commitment, absenteeism, and turnover.* New York: Academic Press.

Mowday, R. T., Steers, R. M., & Porter, L. W. (1979). The measure of organizational commitment. *Journal of Vocational Behavior, 14*, 224–247.

Mumford, A. (1995). Learning styles and mentoring. *Industrial and Commercial Training, 27*(8), 4–7.

Neary, M., Phillips, R., & Davies, B. (1994). *The practitioner-teacher: A study in the introduction of mentors in the Pre-registration Nurse Education Programme in Wales*. Cardiff, Wales: School of Education, University of Wales. Cited in Andrews, M., & Chilton, F. (2000). Student and mentor perceptions of mentoring effectiveness. *Nurse Education Today, 20,* 555–562.

Noe, R. A. (1988). An investigation of the determinants of successful assigned mentoring relationships. *Personnel Psychology, 41*(3), 457–479.

Opipari-Arrigan, L., Stark, L., & Drotar, D. (2005). Benchmarks for work performance of pediatric psychologists. *Journal of Pediatric Psychology, 31,* 630–642.

Organ, D. W., & Konovsky, M. (1989). Cognitive versus affective determinants of organizational citizenship behavior. *Journal of Applied Psychology, 74,* 157–164.

Organ, D. W., & Ryan, K. (1995). A meta-analytic review of attitudinal and dispositional predictors of organizational citizenship behaviors. *Personnel Psychology, 48,* 775–802.

Pfeffer, J. (1981). *Power in organizations*. Marshfield, MA: Pitman.

Podsakoff, P. M., Mackenzie, S. B., & Hui, C. (1993). Organizational citizenship behaviors and managerial evaluations of employee performance: A review and suggestions for future research. *Research in Personnel and Human Resources Management, 11,* 1–40.

Ponce, A. N., Williams, M. K., & Allen, G. J. (2005). Toward promoting generative cultures of intentional mentoring within academic settings. *Journal of Clinical Psychology, 61,* 1159–1163.

Price, J. H., Dake, J. A., & Islam, R. (2001). Selected ethical issues in research and publication: Perceptions of health education faculty. *Health Education & Behavior, 28*(1), 51–64.

Pulsford, D., Boit, K., & Owen, S. (2002). Are mentors ready to make a difference? A survey of mentors' attitudes towards nurse education. *Nurse Education Today, 22*(6), 439–446.

Ragins, B. R. (1997). Antecedents of diversified mentoring relationships. *Journal of Vocational Behavior, 51,* 90–109.

Ragins, B. R., & McFarkin, D. B. (1990). Perceptions of mentor roles in cross-gender mentoring relationships. *Journal of Vocational Behavior, 37,* 321–339.

Ragins, B. R., & Scandura, T. A. (1999). Burden or blessing? Expected costs and benefits of being a mentor. *Journal of Organizational Behavior, 20,* 493–509.

Ragins, B. R., & Sundstrom, E. (1989). Gender and power in organizations: A longitudinal perspective. *Psychological Bulletin, 105,* 51–88.

Ramanan, R. A., Phillips, R. S., Davis, R. B., Silen, W., & Reede, J. Y. (2002). Mentoring in medicine: Keys to satisfaction. *American Journal of Medicine, 112,* 336–341.

Ramani, S. (2006). Twelve tips to promote excellence in medical teaching. *Medical Teacher, 28*(1), 19–23.

Rosenthal, S. L., & Black, M. M. (2006). Commentary—Mentoring—Benchmarks for performance. *Journal of Pediatric Psychology, 31,* 643–646.

Sadler-Smith, E., & Riding, R. J. (1999). Cognitive style and instructional preferences. *Instructional Science, 27,* 355–371.

Scandura, T. A., & Schriesheim, C. A. (1991). Effects of structural characteristics of mentoring dyads on protégé career outcomes. In D. F. Ray & M. E. Schnake (Eds.), *Proceedings of the Southern Management Association* (pp. 206–208). Mississippi State, MS: Southern Management Association.

Shea, G. F. (1999). *Making the most of being mentored*. Boston, MA: Course Technology.

Steers, R. M., & Braunstein, D. N. (1976). A behaviorally based measure of manifest needs in work settings. *Journal of Vocational Behavior, 9*, 251–266.

Stewart, S., & Carpenter, C. (2009). Electronic mentoring: An innovative approach to providing clinical support. *International Journal of Therapy and Rehabilitation, 16*(4), 199–206.

Spitzmüller, C., Neumann, E., Spitzmüller, M., Rubino, C., Keeton, K. E., Sutton, M. T., et al. (2008). Assessing the influence of psychosocial and career mentoring on organizational attractiveness. *International Journal of Selection and Assessment, 16*(4), 403–415.

Suen, L. K. P., & Chow, F. L. W. (2001). Students' perceptions of the effectiveness of mentors in an undergraduate nursing programme in Hong Kong. *Journal of Advanced Nursing, 36*(4), 505–511.

Tennant, M. (1988). *Psychology and adult learning*. London: Routledge.

Tracy, E. E., Jagsi, R., Starr, R., & Tarbell, N. J. (2004). Outcomes of a pilot faculty mentoring program. *American Journal of Obstetrics and Gynecology, 191*, 1846–1850.

Triandis, H. C. (1960). Cognitive similarity and communication in a dyad. *Human Relations, 13*, 175–183.

Walker, W. O., Kelly, P. C., & Hume, R. F., Jr. (2002). Mentoring for the new millennium. *Medical Education Online, 7*, 1–5. Retrieved May 24, 2010, from http://www.med-ed-online.org

Watty, K. (2003). When will academics learn about quality? *Quality in Higher Education, 9*(3), 213–221.

Wingard, D. L., Garman, K. A., & Reznik, V. (2004). Facilitating faculty success: Outcomes and cost benefit of the UCSD National Center of Leadership in Academic Medicine. *Academic Medicine, 79*(10), S9–S11.

Witkin, H. A., & Goodenough, D. R. (1981). *Cognitive style: Essence and origins*. New York: International Universities Press.

Witkin, H. A., Moore, C. A., Goodenough, D. R., & Cox, P. W. (1977). Field dependent and field independent cognitive styles and their educational implications. *Review of Educational Research, 47*(1), 1–64.

Wright-Harp, W., & Cole, P. A. (2008). A mentoring model for enhancing success in graduate education. *Contemporary Issues in Science and Disorders, 35*, 4–16.

Zachary, L. J. (2000). *The mentor's guide*. Hoboken, NJ: Jossey-Bass.

FIVE

Case Study Five

Evaluation of the Mentor–Mentee Relationship

Eric Rice and Oscar Grusky

INTRODUCTION

Mentorship is a critical part of the training of the next generation of academics in the health and behavioral sciences. This chapter uses the coauthors' mentor–mentee relationship as a case study for the purposes of exploring and evaluating what constitutes a successful mentor–mentee relationship. This case study describes the relationship between a senior scientist and a postdoctoral fellow. Dr. Grusky (the mentor), a senior scientist, is research professor in the School of Public Affairs at UCLA. He has been the director of many NIH research training programs and has been, and currently serves as, director of an AIDS research training program funded by the National Institute of Mental Health (NIMH) since 1989 where he has mentored 75 predoctoral and postdoctoral fellows. He is also a member of the Council of Advisors at the University of California Los Angeles (UCLA), a group that provides junior faculty members with career advice. Dr. Rice (the mentee) was a postdoctoral fellow in Dr. Grusky's program; following the completion of his fellowship, he was appointed for 5 years as a research sociologist in the UCLA Semel Institute for Neuroscience and Human Behavior. This chapter begins with a description of our conceptual model, followed by the presentation of a particular case and a discussion of the evidence and its limitations, and concludes with comments on future directions.

THE MODEL

The Mentor–Mentee Relationship as a Source of Reciprocal Social Support

Mentoring is defined as an evolving social interactive process that ideally helps mentees to become independent scholars or, more generally, to become leaders in their chosen field of work and also enables mentors to become life-long advisors and friends to the next generation of intellectual innovators. A number of students opt for an academic career and, like every career, this choice means struggling and confronting numerous social stressors, ranging from pressures to publish, to teach effectively, to win grants, and to secure honors, positions, and promotions. It is empirically well-established that social support mitigates the negative impact of stress and improves the health of individuals (Berkman & Syme, 1979; Cohen & Wills, 1985; House, Landis, & Umberson, 1988). An effective mentor–mentee relationship is one of mutual social support, including instrumental, emotional, and informational support. In large part, the relationship mitigates stress insofar as it is typically focused on problem solving and task accomplishment, which in the context of a supportive working relationship increases the successful attainment of important career milestones and reduces uncertainty, thereby reducing stress.

A successful mentor–mentee relationship is one in which there is a reciprocal flow of social support within the context of the mentor–mentee dyad. To use the language of social exchange theory, an effective mentor–mentee dyad should be a reciprocal exchange relationship (Blau, 1964; Cook & Emerson, 1978; Emerson, 1962, 1972, 1981; Homans, 1961; Molm, Peterson, & Takahashi, 1999). A positive and enduring mentor–mentee relationship is one where both parties receive valued social goods from one another. Social exchange theorists have pointed out that when social exchange relationships become unbalanced, when the give and take of those relations is uneven, relations tend to deteriorate. When an exchange relationship is well-balanced, that is, when both parties are actively engaged in the give and take of valued social goods, that relationship can endure for years, if not a lifetime (Blau, 1964; Molm et al., 1999). In a successful mentor–mentee relationship, both parties are at least tacitly aware of the benefits and responsibilities of their side of the relationship that lead to the giving and receiving of instrumental, informational, and emotional support.

Benefits and Responsibilities of the Mentor–Mentee Relationship

(Mentee) The benefits to the mentee of the mentor–mentee relationship are many. The following list is likely incomplete, but it should provide the reader with a sense of the core issues. Mentees are often the recipients of financial support in the form of fellowships, research assistantships, or teaching assistantships. The mentee is typically the recipient of career guidance from the more experienced mentor, ranging from formal training plans to informal career discussions. The mentee benefits from the established mentor's status, prestige, and network of collaborators. Early in a mentee's career, prior to producing a body of work of one's own, the mentor provides the mentee with an identity as a student of a successful academic. Later in a mentee's career, this social status can be useful in obtaining fellowships and in securing employment. The mentor's collaborators may include other faculty in a department and worldwide, community-based organizations, program officers at granting institutions, and other mentees. In all cases, the pathways to new collaborations are easier to traverse because of the mentor's existing social ties to these key players. These key players lead to potential connections with other useful persons and organizations through what social network theorists call the strength of "weak" ties (Granovetter, 1973). Granovetter found that indirect (weak) social connections (friends of friends) can yield even greater benefits in job-seeking than direct (strong) ties. The mentee is often the recipient of invaluable hands-on training opportunities in the form of collaborative manuscript writing, data analysis, field work, and grant writing. The mentee often benefits from emotional support from the mentor. The process of establishing a successful career is a stressful one and the mentee can often find the care and kindness one needs to persevere through adversities in the office of a committed mentor. There is no substitute for experience, and within academia most of that experience comes in graduate school and in postdoctoral training in the context of a strong and supportive mentor–mentee relationship.

As with any reciprocal relationship, there are several key responsibilities attendant to the role of mentee. It is the responsibility of the mentee to treat the mentor with respect, not out of blind obedience to seniority, but rather in deference to the commitment inherent in the relationship. It is the mentee's responsibility to work hard. This is perhaps the most important responsibility incumbent in the role, as one's diligent and self-motivated labors are one of the greatest resources a mentee has to offer in the relationship. It is the mentee's responsibility to listen to the mentor with an open mind. By definition, the mentor has substantial experience, and while a mentor cannot have all the answers, he or she likely has some or many. It is the responsibility of the mentee to maintain open and honest communication with the mentor. Mentors are fallible humans and may not always perceive the full impact that their actions and words may have on a mentee (both good and bad). The mentee should seek to communicate with the mentor their personal perspectives on an issue.

(Mentor) The mentor is obligated to do what he/she can to help the mentee become an independent and innovative scholar, for example, by helping the mentee develop needed skills and by providing a training environment that advances the mentee's career. The responsibilities of the mentor vis-à-vis the mentee start ideally with the obligation to serve as an example in every possible way. The term "ideally" is used because human beings are imperfect, so both the mentor and mentee may on occasion fail to meet their respective responsibilities. If that happens, and the relationship is based on mutual trust, there should be mutual understanding such that even failure can function to strengthen the relationship. One-on-one teaching works best when the mentor-teacher represents through his or her actions, as well as through his or her words, the kinds of behavior that are appropriate to the situation. It is the mentor's responsibility to do his/her best to develop mutual support, trust, and respect in the relationship with the mentee. The mentor should help the mentee develop as an ethical scholar/teacher/researcher by making himself/herself readily available should any issues requiring advice arise. It is the duty and the responsibility of the mentor to be as accessible and as constructive (i.e., focused on problem-solving) as possible.

The benefits that accrue to the mentor are the gains that accrue to all teachers including the personal rewards of learning from the mentee new ways of looking at issues and the opportunity to help shape and inform a young scholar. Perhaps among the greatest rewards of mentoring are the pride one obtains from contributing even in small ways to the development and successes of the mentee.

THE CASE

Focal Training Issues as Seen by the Mentor and the Mentee

In this section, we examine three focal training issues as seen by the mentee and the mentor. Each of these issues is a pivotal component of postdoctoral training. The issues are developing a training plan, issues in producing publications, and issues in getting an academic job. We assume that at the very outset of the mentor–mentee relationship, there is an explicit or implicit contract between them. That contract contains elements such as the commitment of the institution to train the mentee by meeting the highest possible professional standards, a focus on encouraging the mentee to become an independent scholar, to uphold the highest standards of ethical conduct and professional responsibility in research and teaching, and to foster a shared mutual respect for one another as individuals.

Creating a Plan for a 2-Year Postdoctoral Fellowship

(Mentee) Being mentored in the creation of a specific plan for my 2 year postdoctoral fellowship was critical to my success in that program. This task was especially important in my case as my graduate training, while in sociology, was in neither medical sociology nor behavioral issues in HIV/AIDS. I took this postdoctoral fellowship with the explicit intention of moving away from the experimental and theoretical social psychology training I had received in graduate school, and moving into the field of behavioral research on HIV/AIDS. Two years was a short time, indeed, for such an ambitious goal.

The plan, itself, was born from a series of meetings I had with the mentor. He rightly insisted that I create a concrete written plan for my goals across the 2 years that I would be a fellow under him, and that I work out in detail what my specific tasks would be especially for the first year. After our initial meeting, it was clear that the most important task was finding a specific mentor who worked in the area in which I wanted to gain expertise. My plan hinged on getting involved in a working research group immediately, so that I could begin to work on research projects and papers in the area of HIV prevention. It was my belief, and one supported by the mentor, that there was no substitute for hands-on training through collaboration with senior scientists in my newly chosen area of concentration.

To locate a mentor in the area of HIV prevention, I availed myself of the network of scientific collaborators which the mentor had. I set up initial meetings to discuss the possibilities of collaborating with about a half dozen senior scholars doing work in the field. At the time, I believed that some of these meetings had been more promising than others, but my opinions were based largely on this one face-to-face meeting. So back to the mentor I went, now armed with these first impressions, to seek his advice on which of these scholars would be the best mentor to me.

The mentor is not a man afraid to share his opinions with his mentees, which is something I have always appreciated about him. I do not always agree with him, but at least I can form an opinion either in agreement or in opposition to him. There is nothing worse in a mentor than a lack of guidance. In this case, I will be forever grateful to the mentor's opinions. When I returned with my list of scholars and reported on my meetings with each of them, the mentor immediately and vehemently recommended one scholar in particular, who in his opinion was far senior, a more successful grant winner, and more highly published than the rest. He believed that although I could do well under the mentorship of many of the others I met, none would provide me with the experience and guidance offered by Dr. Rotheram. In the end, my time in her research center as a postdoctoral fellow and then as a staff researcher for the following 5 years helped establish my initial career successes.

(Mentor) All of my predoctoral ("predocs") and postdoctoral ("postdocs") trainees in my NIMH AIDS research training program are asked to produce a detailed plan for each year of their research training. I work closely with each trainee both on the initial draft of their plan and on the changes that are made to their initial and succeeding drafts. The plan typically consists of several parts:

1. Career goals—academic/nonacademic/other or to be determined. This consists of a brief statement where the mentee explains his/her long term career goals;
2. Major current areas of research interest. This consists of a description of the mentee's main research interests including a specification of the work they are currently doing and/or plan on completing the coming academic year;
3. Required courses/experiences for the training program. The training program requires a number of courses in several departments and has several research experience requirements. In this section, the mentee provides for the Fall, Winter, and Spring Quarter his/her specific plan for fulfilling each of these requirements;
4. Required courses/experiences for the predoc's PhD program or desired/needed special courses for postdoctoral fellows. This is self-explanatory;
5. Specialized courses in areas of interest. This is also self-explanatory;
6. Community based organization (CBO) experiences. The mentee describes his/her plan for meeting the program's community-based organization experience requirement. This involves spending a period of time evaluating a CBO program that the CBO wants evaluated;
7. Presentations at conferences and other professional development experiences, including a required research presentation at the annual Center for HIV Intervention Prevention and Treatment Services (CHIPTS) "HIV: The Next Generation" Conference;
8. Preparation of a list of potential HIV scientific mentors; and
9. Other areas of interest such as taking specialized advanced methods courses or teaching in areas of interest.

The overall goal of the training program is to assist the trainee to become an independent scholar in HIV/AIDS research by fostering a high-quality research training experience. The quality of the mentoring is of obvious importance to achieving the goal. There are 24 professors/mentors in the UCLA program, and they are selected not only because of the quality of their scholarship but also because of their ability to mentor by being available to their mentees, offering their guidance, sharing knowledge, and encouraging the student's development.

Obviously, many considerations are involved in selecting an appropriate mentor. One is whether or not the two parties wish to work together. Do their interests gel? Do they get along with one another? Do they both define their relationship in positive terms? Is the mentor too busy to take on another student? The mentor must agree to complete a brief formal quarterly evaluation of the mentee's performance. Professor Rotheram is a brilliant HIV scholar, runs several programs and centers, is internationally known, and is extraordinarily busy, so she is unable to take on large numbers of mentees. However, it was evident that the mentee and Rotheram had similar intellectual interests, and I hoped and anticipated that their "chemistry" would be good, as indeed it turned out to be. (Needless to say, this prediction sometimes is wrong.) Since she is exceptionally busy the trade-off was that the smaller amount of time might be available, but the high quality of that time together would more than make-up for the quantity. Consequently, I recommended that the mentee consider Dr. Rotheram as his mentor and both parties consented.

Writing Manuscripts Collaboratively

(Mentee) In large measure, what has led to the successful generation of this particular piece is the dynamic interplay of ideas flowing across our mentor–mentee relationship. As the mentor explains in the following section, the organization and thrust of this chapter shifted over time. While he is generous in attributing most of this shift to my contribution, I believe that the final format we are taking to the writing of this piece emerged from the relationship. Despite his coming to our initial meeting about this paper with a well-formulated model and set of organizational ideas about the manuscript, the meeting quickly became a very organic discussion about the dyadic nature of the mentor–mentee relationship. We were both quite taken with the idea that despite the inherent power differentials in such a relationship, there is a genuine reciprocity in productive mentor–mentee relationships.

After our first meeting regarding the manuscript, I left with the task of outlining much of what we had discussed, which at that point still included a heavy focus on the mentor's initial conceptual model. To be perfectly frank, the resulting outline was boring and pedantic. When we next met and poured over this labored first attempt, I raised the concern that we had not focused enough on a specific case or set of cases. The mentor agreed and we then laid out a very different approach that focused on a set of positive and negative cases we had each experienced. As I began to write, I found myself writing mostly about our successful mentor–mentee relationship because I wanted to describe the workings of a successful mentor–mentee relationship. Moreover, I found it difficult to write about negative mentoring experiences without coming across as blaming or without recounting potentially embarrassing moments in the history of my mentor–mentee relationships. These "horror" story anecdotes, while true, may have painted mentors for whom I have deep respect and admiration in an overly negative light which

I felt did not reflect the true overall quality and depth of those relationships. When we met a third time, we settled on the current format.

One of the positive side effects of working on manuscripts together is that it provides an opportunity for the mentor and mentee to discuss not just the work in question but also other ideas, career aspirations, and life in general. Working on this manuscript has been no exception. The timing of this manuscript has coincided with my pursuit of a tenure track academic appointment. Our meetings over the past months which were ostensibly to work on the manuscript were devoted at least as much to support with respect to my job search as to work on the chapter. Although the timing of my job search and the nature of this manuscript have made both of us more self-conscious of the process and our relationship, I think that support around multiple aspects of one's career is more often than not an ongoing part of mentor–mentee collaborations.

(Mentor) In discussing this topic of publications, the mentee and I started out sharing stories about those rare cases (in our experiences, at least) where the relationships not only did not pan out but were disastrous. We agreed, however, that it would be far better to focus on successful collaborations. We both consider our collaboration on this chapter a successful one. When the editor of this book first approached me about writing a chapter, I accepted with the idea of writing it myself, in part, perhaps, because I had single-authored a chapter in a book that she published in 2007. However, once I started thinking about the topic and the model(s) that were likely to be used, I felt the need for a mentee as a collaborator, since a collaborative approach would greatly increase the likelihood that the chapter would better reflect the perspectives and insights of both parties. The editor agreed, and so I asked the mentee to be coauthor and he accepted. When he and I started discussing the chapter, I already had a potential model that I described and that the mentee liked, and so we both implicitly assumed that I would be first author and he would be second author. However, the mentee soon came up with a number of excellent ideas for restructuring the chapter. In light of these ideas, I proposed that we reverse roles and that he be the first author. This example reveals the evolving nature of a collaborative writing project. It also implies the significant role of understanding and mutual respect in collaborative endeavors. More generally, it demonstrates the need for good communication leading to understanding and mutual respect in the mentor–mentee relationship.

Searching for an Academic Position

(Mentee) Trying to land my first job as an assistant professor has been a stressful task and one which I could not have navigated successfully without the assistance of several key mentors. When I initially decided that

I was ready to pursue an academic appointment, I first went to the mentor who had been my advisor during my postdoctoral fellowship 5 years earlier. I had received consistently solid mentoring from the mentor over the past few years, and I knew that he could provide me with guidance in this process, given his successful track record of helping many other mentees over the years accomplish the same goal.

At our initial meeting, the mentor provided me with constructive feedback about how to approach the job search. He advised that if I were to get a job, I would need to conduct a nationwide search and apply to every job in which my research portfolio fit. In my case, my work bridges three types of departments/schools: schools of public health, schools of social work, and sociology departments interested in applied medical sociology. As such, I had my work cut out for me because I needed to come up with three slightly different approaches to my job search.

After our initial meeting, during which the mentor helped me to brainstorm the types of positions that I might seek out, he set me to the invaluable task of writing a summary statement of my teaching, research, grant writing, and community-based experiences from which he could write his letters of support for me. My first pass at this task was a disaster. The mentor, in his usual unflinching style, told me exactly what worked (very little) and what did not (quite a lot). His extensive feedback to this initial draft formed the basis of my subsequent revisions. In the end, I had a clear and concise description of my teaching interests, my research agenda, my history of grant winning, and my commitment to community-based participatory research.

He then provided me with valuable feedback about how many departments to focus on—including a cautionary tale about a former mentee who had applied to more than 100 jobs! He quite rightly pointed out that there would only be a couple dozen jobs for which I would be a strong candidate. Even this modest number was difficult to manage. In the end, most of my opportunities for interviews came from that handful of departments, where my research agenda was a tight fit with the parameters of the search. The jobs that were on the margins, in the end, were probably not worth my energy.

The mentor's guidance around the job search extended to writing letters on my behalf, talking to interested departments, and advocating for me. When it finally came time for me to take my first trip out of town to deliver a job talk, the mentor arranged a mock job talk session for me. He invited some of his colleagues and other mentees to my practice job talk, attended by eight people, including a postdoctoral fellow who had gotten a job at a top school of social work 1 year earlier, another faculty member, two graduate students, and two staff researchers. With their invaluable feedback, I was able to revamp my job talk with respect to pace, focus more on my theory, and provide a more detailed and compact discussion of my central results. This moved me away from unfinished work, focusing instead on work that was more complete and polished.

In the end, I gave my job talk at five schools/departments, and I received three formal job offers and one informal offer. I accepted a position as a tenure track assistant professor at the School of Social Work of the University of Southern California (USC). In the 3 months between my initial practice job talk and when I accepted USC's offer, the mentor was a continual source of good advice. As I returned from each trip, he would counsel me on how to engage with faculty at the various institutions, so that I would be in a prime position to receive formal (and written) offers. And, perhaps most importantly, he and my other mentors provided me with many recommendations and personal encouragement all along the way.

In addition to the mentor, I received invaluable mentoring, support and advice from Dr. Norweeta Milburn, Dr. Mary Jane Rotheram, and Dr. Steve Shoptaw. Triangulating mentors' advice around the job search is critical. Most academics, whether intentionally or not, will advise mentees to follow a path similar to their career path or what they wish they had pursued. To find a balanced view of job opportunities, I have found it useful to discuss my options with many different senior scientists who were willing to mentor me.

(Mentor) Obviously getting an academic position is largely dependent on the scholar's academic abilities, but one should never underestimate the relevance of careful preparation, strategic decision making, and the ability to mobilize and apply effectively one's interpersonal skills. I have learned a great deal from studying organizational behavior for many years, from studying organizations and teaching organization theory, from running a business, creating new organizations, supervising and helping to place predocs and postdocs, and chairing a large academic department.

Some students on the academic job market for the first time may be unaware that a key element in getting an academic position is actually obtaining a written job offer. Accordingly, I advised the mentee of the value and importance of going beyond a verbal job offer and obtaining a written job offer ("sealing the deal"). This may seem obvious to some applicants, but it is often not obvious to others. A letter is needed to help reduce the uncertainty that is built-into the situation. The primary reason for requesting an offer in writing is to avoid misunderstandings. Some candidates confuse a verbal offer with a written offer, and occasionally that can lead to undesirable misunderstandings. I did not want the mentee to make that mistake. This is a touchy issue since the first-time job applicant does not want to appear "pushy" or be perceived by the department chair as someone who does not trust the chair. The chair, on the other hand, does not want to have to report to her/his dean that the proffered offer was rejected. Hence, the chair may want verbal acceptance of a job offer prior to providing a written offer while the candidate may be understandably concerned that the offer in writing may not be the same as the verbal offer.

A second issue on which I sought to help the mentee concerned focusing on the essential difference between a 9-month academic ladder position and a part-time ladder position. The mentee was an applicant for two posts, one of each type, in the same large academic organization. Naturally, he was totally above-board and informed both units about his application for a position in the other unit. Nevertheless, a tactical dilemma was created by his being wooed by two different units in the same university, which was a topic of discussion between us. That dilemma was created by the different character of the two positions. A proposed solution was to define one position (the 9-month position) as more central and desirable than the other and to consider the other one as less central and worth considering only as a supplementary post.

EVALUATION

One of the principal limitations of this study and of all case studies of this kind is selection bias. Selection bias takes place when it is not possible to sample the entire range of values on an outcome variable (Berk, 1983). If only successful mentor–mentee dyads are studied and failures are obscured, then we may be unlikely to gain understanding of the mechanisms associated with either success or failure because of lack of a comparison group. This case, however, provides a good example of a successful relationship, even if that success cannot be generalized to the whole population of mentor–mentee dyads.

This mentor–mentee relationship was successful with respect to all three of the core tasks aforementioned: creating a plan for a 2-year postdoctoral position, collaborative writing, and searching for an academic position. All three tasks have distinct outcomes that can be cited as measures of success. The mentor helped the mentee successfully find an HIV prevention mentor with whom to work, which led the mentee to seven successful years of publishing and grant writing. The mentor and the mentee successfully collaborated on this chapter and hopefully, the reader has found it illuminating and thought-provoking. Finally, the mentor successfully supported the mentee in his search for and appointment to a tenure track faculty position at a major research university. It is notable that two of the three outcomes are focused primarily on the outcomes of the mentee, but it is important to remember that in a well-functioning mentor–mentee relationship, the mentee's successes are a reflection of his/her mentoring and hence are successes for the mentor as well.

The successful giving and receiving of social support across the mentor–mentee relationship was key to the reduction of stress and the success of the outcomes reported. In the example of the mentee's search for a senior HIV prevention scientist with whom to work, the mentor provided a great deal of social support. He provided instrumental support in the form of his specific network ties which the mentee could draw upon to secure introductory meetings with other scientists; financial support in the form of the 2 years of postdoctoral funding; and informational support during the period of uncertainty surrounding the mentee's selection process. The financial support allowed the mentee to work with senior scientists in the field of HIV prevention research, and the informational support provided the mentee with additional information about each of the scientists, with whom the mentee was considering working, thereby allowing the mentee to make a more informed decision. Because the creation of a successful postdoctoral plan is a stressful event, the instrumental and informational support often came with more tacit emotional support during the mentee's meetings with the mentor.

Social support is not merely given by the mentor and received by the mentee, although this is often the case. A successful mentor–mentee relationship is characterized by reciprocity. The creation of this manuscript is an example of this reciprocity. The mentor invited the mentee to be a coauthor; during the course of the discussions around the manuscript new ideas emerged from the mentee and the decision was made to shift the focus of the manuscript as well as authorship to the mentee as lead. The mentee, being at an early stage in his career, benefited from the opportunity to be lead author on a chapter, and the mentor benefited from the ideas and efforts put forth by the mentee in the writing of the chapter. Both the mentor and the mentee also took seriously their respective responsibilities in the creation of the manuscript. The mentor provided initial guidance, ongoing encouragement, text, and editorial suggestions, while the mentee provided new direction and focus, drafted much of the manuscript, and provided editorial suggestions. The reciprocity inherent in collaborative manuscript writing is self-evident. The mentor–mentee relationship as a whole must be one of balance and reciprocity for it to endure over time.

Because the approach favored in this study focused almost entirely on symmetry and balance in the mentor–mentee relationship, another study limitation is the failure of the analysis to adequately consider the implications of asymmetric power in the mentor–mentee dyad. For example, consider Emerson's concept of power and how Emerson considered that power and dependency might enter into the mentor–mentee relationship (Emerson, 1962, 1972). Emerson's model emphasized how the mentor and mentee may be tied to one another through dependence or mutual dependence. The dependence of the mentee on the mentor is directly proportional to the mentee's motivational investment in goals that the mentor mediates and is inversely proportional to the availability of these goals to the mentee outside the mentor–mentee dyad. The dependence of the mentee on the mentor serves as the basis for the mentor's power over the mentee. If the mentee cannot do without the resources and cannot get them somewhere else, then to that extent, the mentee is dependent on the mentor. However, the goal of the dyad is to foster independence on the part of the mentee. How can dependence in a relationship actually lead to (evolve into) independence?

Blau's (1964) classic treatment of exchange relationships provides a partial answer. Blau acknowledged that numerous reciprocal relationships indeed have power imbalances as a part of their dynamic. However, he pointed out that imbalances in power in ongoing relationships provide the impetus for social change. Blau argued that people who are in a position of lesser social power experience a certain "hardship" from this experience and strive to escape such relations, staying in them only when to do so outweighs the "hardships" of dependence. So to extend Blau's thinking to the mentor–mentee dyad, the mentee, while initially deriving a great number of social rewards from the relationship, is likely over time to feel more "hardship" from dependence as the mentee develops an increasingly successful independent career. So the very dependence that makes the relationship function also generates the impetus for the mentee to move on. This is not to suggest that the mentor–mentee relationship is one of great imbalance. Mentors are dependent upon mentees to successfully and diligently work to provide support to their joint academic work (as we discussed earlier). The point we wish to make is that the imbalances that exist provide some of the impetus for mentees to grow and move away from any particular mentoring relationship over time as they become increasingly independent. A mentor–mentee relationship which is enduring over a lifetime is apt to become increasingly a relationship of equals, where power imbalances lessen over time. This is facilitated by both parties' initiatives and both parties' willingness and desire to encourage independence.

FUTURE DIRECTIONS FOR THE MENTOR–MENTEE RELATIONSHIP

We have described a case of a successful mentor–mentee relationship built upon the reciprocal exchange of social support over time. Because it is a relatively balanced mentor–mentee relationship we anticipate that it will continue for years to come. An example of the ongoing nature of this mentor–mentee relationship emerged from a meeting that took place as we were finishing writing this chapter.

(Mentee) Once I accepted my tenure track position, after warmly and enthusiastically congratulating me, the mentor asked about the details of my new position and the expectations for tenure incumbent to this post. I reported that the most difficult and most important marker for success in my new position as defined specifically by the institution will be winning an NIH R01 grant, which is no small task. We spent the better part of the next hour discussing different routes for successfully obtaining an R01 in the behavioral sciences, focusing in particular on the importance of work integrating new technologies into my work on HIV risks in the social networks of homeless youth. It is hard to imagine that this relationship will end with my leaving for this new position. Instead the mutual support and collaboration is likely to go on and on.

(Mentor) As part of my experience mentoring, I am aware that helping the mentee get a job as an assistant professor is only the beginning. This is because successful mentees need advice on steps that need to be taken to be promoted to tenure that include how to get grants and expand their social networks and their technological skills. They will need letters of recommendation if considered for other jobs or when considered for promotion to associate professor and then to full professor. And they will definitely need the advice, support, and assistance of multiple mentors.

As a final thought, we suggest that a good mentor–mentee relationship begets the next generation of mentor–mentee relationships, where the mentee becomes the mentor to others in the future. Good mentoring provides a model for future mentoring by the mentee. In the present case, the mentee benefited from several mentors including the mentor who is coauthor. Indeed, the mentee has already begun the process of mentoring others. In particular, the mentee has two former research assistants, who were coauthors with him on his manuscripts, whom he mentored through the process of applying to and successfully becoming accepted at top PhD programs. One of his mentees is currently a student in clinical psychology at Clark University and the other was recently accepted into the PhD program at the School of Social Work at the University of Washington, Seattle. Thus, a successful mentor–mentee relationship not only endures for years, but may also be replicated across future generations.

REFERENCES

Berk, R. A. (1983). An introduction to sample selection bias in sociological data. *American Sociological Review, 48,* 386–398.

Berkman, L. F., & Syme, L. (1979). Social networks, host resistance, and mortality: a nine year follow-up study of Alameda county residents. *American Journal of Epidemiology, 109,* 186–204.

Blau, P. M. (1964). *Exchange and power in social life.* New York: Wiley.

Cohen, S., & Wills, T. A. (1985). Stress social support, and the buffering hypothesis. *Psychological Bulletin, 98,* 310–357.

Cook, K. S., & Emerson, R. M. (1978). Power, equity and commitment in exchange networks. *American Sociological Review, 43,* 721–739.

Emerson, R. M. (1962). Power-dependence relations. *American Sociological Review, 27,* 31–41.

Emerson, R. M. (1972). Exchange theory, part II: Exchange relations and networks. In J. Berger, M. Zelditch Jr., & B. Anderson (Eds.), *Sociological theories in progress* (Vol. 2, pp. 58–87). Boston: Houghton-Mifflin.

Emerson, R. M. (1981). Social exchange theory. In M. Rosenberg & R. H. Turner (Eds.), *Social psychology: Sociological perspectives* (pp. 30–65). New York: Basic Books.

Granovetter, M. S. (1973). The strength of weak ties. *American Journal of Sociology, 78,* 1360–1380.

Homans, G. C. (1961). *Social behaviour: Its elementary forms.* New York: Harcourt, Brace & World.

House, J. S., Landis, K. R., & Umberson, D. (1988). Social relationships and health. *Science, 241,* 540–545.

Molm, L. D., Peterson, G., & Takahashi, N. (1999). Power in negotiated and reciprocal exchange. *American Sociological Review, 64,* 876–890.

Index